Get Th

MRCC Qs and EMQs

Get Through

MRCOG Part 1: MCQs and EMQs

Rekha Wuntakal MBBS MD(O&G) DNB DFFP MRCOG
Specialist Registrar in Obstetrics and Gynaecology, Whipps Cross University Hospital NHS Trust, London

Tony Hollingworth MBChB PhD MBA FRCS(Ed) FRCOG
Consultant in Obstetrics and Gynaecology, Whipps Cross University Hospital NHS Trust, London

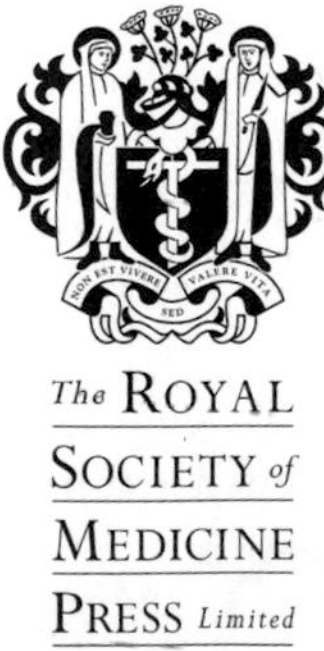

The ROYAL SOCIETY of MEDICINE PRESS Limited

Published by the Royal Society of Medicine Press Ltd
1 Wimpole Street, London W1G 0AE, UK
Tel: +44 (0)20 7290 2921
Fax: +44 (0)20 7290 2929
Email: publishing@rsm.ac.uk
Website: www.rsmpress.co.uk

British Library Cataloguing in Publication Data
A catalogue record for this book is available from the British Library

ISBN: 978-1-85315-971-8

Distribution in Europe and Rest of the World:
Marston Book Services Ltd
PO Box 269
Abingdon
Oxon OX14 4YN, UK
Tel: +44 (0)1235 465500
Fax: +44 (0)1235 465555
Email: direct.order@marston.co.uk

Distribution in the USA and Canada:
Royal Society of Medicine Press Ltd
c/o BookMasters Inc
30 Amberwood Parkway
Ashland, OH 44805, USA
Tel: +1 800 247 6553/+1 800 266 5564
Fax: +1 419 281 6883
Email: order@bookmasters.com

Distribution in Australia and New Zealand:
Elsevier Australia
30-52 Smidmore Street
Marrickville NSW 2204, Australia
Tel: +61 2 9517 8999
Fax: +61 2 9517 2249
Email: service@elsevier.com.au

Typeset by Techset Composition Limited, Salisbury, UK
Printed and bound in Great Britain by Bell & Bain, Glasgow

Mixed Sources
Product group from well-managed forests and other controlled sources
www.fsc.org Cert no. TT-COC-002769
© 1996 Forest Stewardship Council

Contents

Introduction

The Membership of the Royal College of Obstetricians and Gynaecologists (MRCOG) examination can be considered the most important international postgraduate examination in obstetrics and gynaecology. It is divided into two parts. Part 1 of the MRCOG examination examines candidates' knowledge of the basic and applied sciences relevant to the clinical practice of obstetrics and gynaecology. The curriculum is set out in a series of modules which are then divided into a series of domains that look at:

- Understanding cell function
- Understanding human structure
- Understanding measurement and manipulation
- Understanding illness.

This information can be easily accessed through the RCOG website, available at: www.rcog.org.uk.

The examination comprises two papers each lasting 2 hours. The format of both papers is identical, with 20 extended matching questions (EMQs) and 48 '5-part' multiple choice questions (MCQs). There are 60 marks for the EMQs and 240 marks for the MCQs with no negative marking. This results in a mark out of 300 per paper. The pass mark is determined by the Angoff method of standard setting. Standard setting is covered in the RCOG Press publication, *The MRCOG: A guide to the examination*, 3rd edition.

The content of the papers is as follows:

Paper 1 Anatomy, embryology, endocrinology, microbiology/virology, pharmacology, statistics/epidemiology, clinical trial design and analysis.

Paper 2 Biochemistry, molecular and cellular biology, biophysics, genetics, genomics, regulation of gene expression, immunology, pathology and physiology.

The aim of the examination is to assess candidates' understanding of the basic clinical sciences and how they influence and affect clinical practice.

This book sets out MCQs and EMQs that cover the syllabus of the MRCOG Part 1. The examination will have been blue-printed to ensure an even coverage of the subjects and domains in the curriculum and syllabus. This book should therefore be used as an adjunct to your revision, and familiarity with the format of MCQs and EMQs will be important to succeed in the examination. However, this should not be used as a substitute for ensuring adequate preparation of the basic sciences, which will stand one in good stead for clinical practice and the Part 2 examination.

We would like to thank Ms Deepa Janga and Mr Richard Maplethorpe for their contribution to Microbiology and Physics.

Reference

Ledger WL, Murphy MG. *The MRCOG: A guide to the examination*, 3rd edn. London: RCOG Press, 2008.

Recommended reading

Arulkumaran S, Symonds I, Fowlie A. *Oxford handbook of obstetrics and gynaecology*. New York: Oxford University Press, 2004.

Bennett PN, Brown MJ. *Clinical pharmacology*, 10th edn. Edinburgh: Churchill Livingstone, 2008.

Bhatnagar SM, Kothari ML, Mehta LA. *Essentials of human genetics*, 4th edn. Bombay: Orient Longman, 1999.

Bland M. *Introduction to medical statistics*, 3rd edn. New York: Oxford University Press, 2000.

Chard T, Lilford R. *Basic sciences for obstetrics and gynaecology*, 5th edn. New York: Springer, 2000.

de Swiet M, Chamberlain G, Bennett P. *Basic science in obstetrics and gynaecology – a textbook for MRCOG part 1*, 3rd edn. New York: Churchill Livingstone, 2001.

Ganong WF. *Review of medical physiology*, 22nd edn. New York: McGraw-Hill, 2005.

Kingston H. *ABC of clinical genetics*, 3rd edn. London: Wiley-Blackwell, 2002.

Kumar V, Abbas AK, Fausto N, Mitchell R. *Robbins basic pathology*, 8th edn. Philadelphia: Saunders, 2007.

Ledger WL, Murphy MG. *The MRCOG: A guide to the examination*, 3rd edn. London: RCOG Press, 2008.

Murray RK, Granner DK, Mayes P, Rodwell V. *Harper's illustrated biochemistry*, 27th edn. New York: McGraw-Hill, 2006.

RCOG. *Past papers – MRCOG Part 1 multiple choice questions, 1997–2001*. London: RCOG Press, 2004.

Reid JL, Rubin PC, Walters M. *Lecture notes: Clinical pharmacology and therapeutics*, 7th edn. London: Wiley-Blackwell, 2006.

Sadler TW. *Langman's medical embryology*, 11th edn. Philadelphia: Lippincott Williams & Wilkins, 2009.

Sinnatamby CS. *Last's anatomy – regional and applied*, 11th edn. New York: Churchill Livingstone, 2006.

Abbreviations

ACE	angiotensin-converting enzyme
ACTH	adrenocorticotrophic hormone
ADP	adenosine diphosphate
AFP	α-fetoprotein
ANA	antinuclear antibody
APH	antepartum haemorrhage
APS	antiphospholipid antibody syndrome
APTT	activated partial thromboplastin time
ATP	adenosine triphosphate
BCG	Bacillus Calmette–Guérin
BCKDH	branched chain α-ketoacid-dehydrogenase complex
BMI	body mass index
C1	complement 1
C2	complement 2
C3	complement 3
CAH	congenital adrenal hyperplasia
cAMP	adenosine cyclic monophosphate
CEMACH	Confidential Enquiries into Maternal Deaths
cGMP	guanosine cyclic monophosphate
CIN	cervical intraepithelial neoplasia
CK	creatine kinase
CMV	cytomegalovirus
CNS	central nervous system
CoA	coenzyme A
COCP	combined oral contraceptive pill
copper IUD	copper intrauterine contraceptive device
CRH	corticotrophin-releasing hormone
CTPA	computed tomographic pulmonary angiography
CVS	chorionic villus biopsy
DHEA	dehydroepiandrosterone
DHT	dihydrotestosterone
DIC	disseminated intravascular coagulation
DNA	deoxyribonucleic acid
DOPA	3,4-dihydroxyphenylalanine
DUB	dysfunctional uterine bleeding
DVT	deep vein thrombosis
E	early
E2	oestrogen 2 (receptor)
EBV	Epstein–Barr virus
ECG	electrocardiograph
ELISA	enzyme-linked immunosorbent assay
ER	endoplasmic reticulum
FBC	full blood count
FDA	Food and Drug Administration
FDPs	fibrin degradation products
FISH	fluorescence *in situ* hybridization
FSH	follicle-stimulating hormone
G1PUT	galactose-1-phosphate uridyl transferase

G6PD	glucose-6-phosphate dehydrogenase deficiency
GABA	γ-aminobutyric acid
GFR	glomerular filtration rate
GI	gastrointestinal
GnRH	gonadotrophin-releasing hormone
GTP	guanosine triphosphate
GUM	genitourinary medicine
H_2O_2	hydrogen peroxide
HbA	haemoglobin A
HbC	haemoglobin C
HbSS	haemoglobin SS
HBV	hepatitis B virus
hCG	human chorionic gonadotrophin
HDL	high-density lipoprotein
HELLP	haemolysis, elevated liver enzymes and low platelets
HGPRT	hypoxanthine–guanine phosphoribosyl transferase
HIV	human immunodeficiency virus
HMB	heavy menstrual bleeding
HMG-CoA	hydroxymethylglutaryl coenzyme A
hPL	human placental lactogen
HPV	human papillomavirus
HSV	herpes simplex virus
HTLV	human T-cell lymphoma virus
IgG	immunoglobulin G
IL IgM	interleukin immunoglobulin M
IUGR	intrauterine growth retardation
IUS	intrauterine system
KOH	potassium hydroxide
L	late
LBC	liquid-based cytology
LDL	low-density lipoprotein
LH	luteinizing hormone
LLETZ	large loop excision of transformation zone
LPS	lipopolysaccharide
MAO	monoamine oxidase
MHC	histocompatibility complex
MI	mechanical index
MMR	measles, mumps and rubella
MRSA	meticillin-resistant *Staphylococcus aureus*
NAD	nicotinamide adenine dinucleotide
NHS	National Health Service
NICE	National Institute for Health and Clinical Excellence
NK	natural killer
NPV	negative predictive value
OHSS	ovarian hyperstimulation syndrome
OR	odds ratio
ORF	open reading frame
PAPP-A	pregnancy-associated plasma protein A
PCOS	polycystic ovarian syndrome
PCR	polymerase chain reaction
PE	pulmonary embolism

PGE_2	prostaglandin E_2
PGG_2	prostaglandin G_2
PGH_2	prostaglandin H_2
PID	pelvic inflammatory disease
PPH	postpartum haemorrhage
PPV	positive predictive value
PT	prothrombin time
RBC	red blood cell
RDS	respiratory distress syndrome
RNA	ribonucleic acid
RR	relative risk
SERM	selective oestrogen receptor modulator
SHBG	sex hormone-binding globulin
SLE	systemic lupus erythematosus
SRY gene	sex-determining region on Y chromosome
TB	tuberculosis
TCA	tricarboxylic acid cycle
TI	thermal index
TIB	bone thermal index
TIBC	total iron-binding capacity
TIS	soft tissue thermal index
TNF-α	tumour necrosis factor alpha
TRH	thyroid hormone- or thyrotrophin-releasing hormone
TSH	thyroid-stimulating hormone
TT	thrombin time
TZ	transformation zone
uE_3	urinary estriol
$\dot{V}/\dot{Q}$	ventilation–perfusion ratio
VLDL	very-low-density lipoprotein
VRE	vancomycin-resistant enterococcus
VZ	varicella-zoster
WBC	white blood cell count
WHO	World Health Organization

1. Practice MCQs I: Questions

1. **Structures passing over the pelvic brim**
   a. Superior rectal artery
   b. Psoas muscle
   c. Internal iliac artery
   d. Ureters
   e. Superior gluteal artery

2. **Urogenital diaphragm**
   a. Is located superior to the pelvic diaphragm
   b. Is located inferior to the pelvic diaphragm
   c. Anteriorly, it encloses the bladder
   d. Posteriorly, it encloses the deep transverse perineal muscle
   e. Supports the pelvic organs

3. **The boundaries of the ischiorectal fossa**
   a. Perineal skin forms the base of the fossa
   b. Obturator internus is the lateral boundary
   c. Vagina forms the medial boundary
   d. The apex is formed by the deep transverse perineal muscle
   e. Sacrospinous ligament forms the posterior boundary

4. **The following are true about the pudendal canal**
   a. It contains pudendal artery, pudendal vein but not pudendal nerve
   b. It contains pudendal artery, pudendal nerve but not pudendal vein
   c. It runs medial to obturator externus
   d. It runs along the lateral wall of the ischiorectal fossa
   e. It leaves the pelvis via greater sciatic foramen

5. **With regard to the course of the ureters in females**
   a. The right ureter is in close association with the sigmoid colon before it enters the bladder
   b. Both ureters are almost always found at the bifurcation of the common iliac vessels
   c. Both ureters pass over the pelvic brim, along the anterior wall
   d. Both ureters are retroperitoneal all along in their course until the peritoneum is lost towards the inferior end
   e. Both ureters pass superior to the uterine arteries

6. **Ovarian vessels and nerves**
   a. The left ovarian artery arises from the abdominal aorta
   b. The left ovarian vein drains into the right renal vein
   c. The right ovarian vein drains into the inferior vena cava
   d. Ovarian lymphatics drain into the common iliac nodes
   e. Parasympathetic nerve supply to the ovary comes from the vagus nerve

7. **The following structures are attached to the iliac crest**
   a. Iliacus muscle
   b. Sacroiliac ligament
   c. Quadratus lumborum
   d. Lattissimus dorsi
   e. External oblique muscle

8. **The following are branches of the anterior division of the internal iliac artery**
   a. Superior vesical artery
   b. Superior gluteal artery
   c. Inferior vesical artery
   d. Middle rectal artery
   e. Superior sacral artery

9. **The following are true about lymphatic drainage of the pelvic organs**
   a. The urethra drains to the internal iliac nodes
   b. The parametrium drains to the internal iliac nodes
   c. The middle third of the vagina drains to the internal iliac nodes
   d. The bladder drains to the internal iliac nodes
   e. The lower body of the uterus drains to the internal iliac nodes

10. **The following are correct terminologies with regard to the ligaments and peritoneum in the pelvis**
    a. Suspensory ligament of ovary – it connects the ovary to the uterus
    b. Suspensory ligament of ovary – it is a condensation of endopelvic fascia
    c. Round ligament – it runs from the fundus of the uterus to the labia minora
    d. Ovarian ligament – it connects the ovary to the lateral pelvic wall
    e. Mesovarium – the portion of the broad ligament that suspends the ovaries in place

11. **Psoas major (muscle)**
   a. It is the chief flexor muscle of the thigh and trunk
   b. It passes the pelvic brim, along the anterior wall
   c. It passes deep to the inguinal ligament and attaches to the lesser trochanter of the femur
   d. It pulls the thigh towards the body
   e. It is innervated by S2–4

12. **The relation of the abdominal aorta to the surrounding structures**
   a. It runs retroperitoneally along the anterior aspect of vertebrae to the level of L4
   b. At the bifurcation, the inferior vena cava passes anterior to the aorta
   c. The inferior vena cava lies to the right of and slightly anterior to the abdominal aorta
   d. The left renal vein passes anterior to the aorta
   e. The aorta lies posterior to the uncinate process of the pancreas

13. **The relationship of the structures in the popliteal fossa**
   a. The popliteal artery lies lateral to the tibial nerve
   b. The popliteal artery lies medial to the popliteal vein
   c. The popliteal vein lies medial to the sciatic nerve
   d. The tibial nerve lies medial to the popliteal artery
   e. The tibial nerve lies lateral to the popliteal vein

14. **The following are true with regard to the origin of the perineal muscles**
   a. Bulbocavernosus arises from the perineal body
   b. Superficial transverse perineal muscle arises from the perineal body
   c. Deep transverse perineal muscle arises from ischial spines
   d. Deep transverse perineal muscle arises from perineal body
   e. Ischiocavernosus arises from the lateral aspect of the ischial ramus

15. **Contents of inguinal canal**
   a. Round ligament in females
   b. Ilioinguinal nerve in males
   c. Ilioinguinal nerve in females
   d. Vas deferens in males
   e. Seminiferous tubules in males

16. **Boundaries of inguinal canal**
   a. The floor is formed by round ligament
   b. The roof is formed by internal oblique muscle
   c. The anterior wall is formed by aponeurosis of external oblique muscle and internal oblique muscle
   d. External oblique and transversus abdominis muscles form the roof
   e. Conjoint tendon and transversalis fascia form the posterior wall

17. **The following are true with regard to nerve supply of the lower limb**
   a. Femoral nerve supplies the posterior compartment of the thigh
   b. Obturator nerve supplies the medial compartment of the thigh
   c. Tibial nerve supplies the posterior compartment of the thigh
   d. Superficial peroneal nerve supplies the lateral compartment of the thigh
   e. Common peroneal nerve supplies the anterior compartment of the thigh

18. **The nerves and nerve roots supplying the lower limb**
   a. The common peroneal nerve arises from anterior division of L4 to S3
   b. The femoral nerve arises from posterior division of L2 to L4
   c. The tibial nerve arises from posterior division of L4 to S3
   d. The superficial peroneal nerve arises from anterior division of L4 to S3
   e. The obturator nerve arises from anterior division of L2 to L4

19. **The vagina and lymphatic drainage**
   a. The lower third mainly drains into the superficial inguinal lymph nodes
   b. The middle third drains into the external iliac nodes
   c. The upper third mainly drains into the internal iliac nodes
   d. The posterior vagina ultimately drains into the internal iliac nodes
   e. The upper two-thirds of the vagina drain into the deep inguinal nodes

20. **Trisomy 18 shows the following features**
   a. Flexion of hands and fingers
   b. Low-set deformed ears
   c. Congenital heart defects
   d. Micrognathia
   e. Syndactyly

21. **The following are true with regard to fragile X syndrome**
   a. Occurs less commonly in males than females
   b. Is the common cause of learning disabilities in males
   c. Is associated with small ears
   d. Is associated with large chin (prominent jaw)
   e. Is associated with increased head circumference

22. **Turner syndrome**
   a. Is characterized by gonadal dysgenesis
   b. 98% of fetuses with this syndrome are spontaneously aborted
   c. 45XO is the only monosomy compatible with life
   d. Non-dysjunction in female gamete is the cause in 80% of these women
   e. In affected women, 55% are monosomic for X

23. **Non-dysjunction**
   a. May involve autosomes
   b. May involve sex chromosomes
   c. Occurs during the first meiotic division of germ cells
   d. Can occasionally occur during mitosis
   e. Its incidence increases after the age of 35 years

24. **Down syndrome**
   a. 95% of the cases are due to meiotic non-dysjunction
   b. 5% of the cases are due to mitotic non-dysjunction
   c. The incidence at the age of 40 is 1:100
   d. Low incidence of leukaemia is noted in these individuals
   e. After the age of 35 years, nearly all develop Alzheimer's disease

25. **Spermatogenesis involves**
   a. Formation of the acrosome
   b. Condensation of the cytoplasm
   c. Condensation of the nucleus
   d. Shedding of the cytoplasm
   e. Formation of the neck, middle piece and tail

26. **The following are true with regard to early embryonic development (post-conception)**
   a. Days 14–15 – development of primitive streak
   b. Days 24–25 – caudal neuropores would be closed
   c. Days 26–27 – cranial neuropore would be closed
   d. Days 26–27 – upper limb buds appear
   e. Days 22–23 – cranial neuropores open widely

27. **The events that occur by 12 weeks of fetal development (post-conception) include**
   a. Primary ossification centres develop in long bones
   b. Secondary ossification centres develop in skull
   c. Secondary ossification centres develop in long bones
   d. Intestinal loops are withdrawn into the abdominal cavity
   e. Sex of the fetus can be determined by ultrasound

28. **Amniotic fluid**
   a. Is produced by amniotic cells
   b. Is replaced every 10 hours
   c. Prevents adherence of the embryo to the amnion
   d. Fetus drinks around 400 mL of amniotic fluid every day
   e. Fetal urine is added to the amniotic fluid from fifth month

29. **Omphalocele**
   a. Is herniation of abdominal organs through a large umbilical ring
   b. Is not associated with chromosomal abnormalities
   c. May include organs such as liver, spleen and stomach
   d. Is associated with low mortality rate unlike gastroschisis
   e. Is associated with neural tube defects in 40% of the cases

30. **Craniosynostosis is seen in**
   a. Pfeiffer syndrome
   b. Apert syndrome
   c. Jackson–Weiss syndrome
   d. Crouzon syndrome
   e. Hand–foot–genital syndrome

31. **The following structures develop from the ureteric bud**
   a. Ureter
   b. Urethra
   c. Major calyces
   d. Minor calyces
   e. Collecting tubules

32. **Paramesonephric duct**
   a. Caudally, opens into the abdominal cavity
   b. Caudally, it runs lateral to the mesonephric duct before it crosses it
   c. Caudally, it runs medial to the mesonephric duct, after crossing it ventrally
   d. Caudally, it runs laterally to the mesonephric duct, after crossing it
   e. In midline, it fuses with the opposite mesonephric duct

33. **The remnants of mesonephric system in females are**
   a. Epoophoron
   b. Gartner cyst
   c. Suspensory ligament of ovary
   d. Paroophoron
   e. Round ligament of uterus

34. **The following are correctly matched with regard to development of external genitalia in females**
   a. Genital tubercle – mons pubis
   b. Genital folds – labia minora
   c. Genital swellings – labia majora
   d. Urogenital grove – vestibule
   e. Genital swellings – clitoris

35. **Androgen insensitivity syndrome**
   a. Is X-linked dominant condition
   b. External genitalia appear male
   c. Internal genitalia contain female organs
   d. Uterus and tubes are absent
   e. The vagina is short and blind

36. **Neural crest derivatives include**
   a. Odontoblast
   b. Adrenal medulla
   c. Schwann cells
   d. Melanocytes
   e. Arachnoid matter

37. **During the first trimester the placental membrane is composed of (placental membrane – separates maternal and fetal blood)**
   a. Mesenchymal tissue in villous core
   b. Endothelial lining of fetal vessels
   c. Endothelial lining of maternal vessels
   d. Cytotrophoblastic cells
   e. Syncytiotrophoblastic cells

38. **α-Fetoprotein (AFP)**
   a. Is produced by fetal liver
   b. Maternal serum levels decline after 30 weeks of pregnancy
   c. Amniotic fluid levels decrease if associated with fetal trisomy 18
   d. Maternal serum levels increase if associated with Down syndrome
   e. Amniotic fluid levels increase if associated with fetal bladder extrophy

39. **Prolactin**
   a. Is a polypeptide
   b. Is evolutionarily not related to growth hormone
   c. Is structurally related to thyroid hormone
   d. Is structurally related to growth hormone
   e. High levels inhibit pulsatile GnRH secretion

40. **The following promote prolactin secretion**
   a. Vasopressin
   b. Oxytocin
   c. Dopamine
   d. Vasoactive intestinal peptide
   e. Thyrotrophin-releasing hormone

41. Physiological causes of raised prolactin are
a. Bulimia nervosa
b. Nipple stimulation
c. Anorexia nervosa
d. Pregnancy
e. Renal failure

42. Drugs that are not used in the treatment of hyperprolactinaemia
a. Cabergoline
b. Metoclopramide
c. Quinagolide
d. L-Dopa
e. Bromocriptine

43. Regarding oxytocin and its analogue Syntocinon
a. Oxytocin is produced in the posterior pituitary
b. Prolonged exposure to Syntocinon causes down-regulation of oxytocin receptors
c. Oxytocin inhibits prolactin secretion
d. Oxytocin stimulates contraction of the myoepithelial cells in the breast
e. Prolonged infusion of Syntocinon can cause hyponatraemia

44. With regard to development of secondary sexual characteristics (males and females)
a. Breast growth in females usually begins between 9 and 13 years of age
b. Breast development occurs in three stages
c. Increase in the size of testes is the first sign of puberty in boys
d. The growth spurt in boys usually starts 24 months after the increase in the testicular volume
e. The appearance of pubic hair follows the appearance of breast buds in females

45. With respect to androgen production in females
a. They are produced by both ovaries and adrenal gland
b. DHEA is mainly derived from the adrenal gland
c. Two-thirds of the daily testosterone production is of adrenal origin
d. Androgens are excreted predominantly as 17-oxogenic steroids after metabolism
e. Androgens exert their effect by binding to intracellular receptors

46. **With regard to gonadotrophins (FSH and LH)**
   a. The half-life of luteinizing hormone is 90 minutes
   b. LH has a shorter half-life than FSH
   c. The half-life of FSH is twice that of LH
   d. Less frequent pulses cause no change in the LH and increase in the FSH
   e. They are released every 60 minutes during the follicular phase

47. **Enzymes involved in synthesis of steroid hormones in females**
   a. The enzyme 21-hydroxylase is required to convert 17-hydroxypregnenolone to 11-deoxycortisol
   b. 11β-Hydroxysteroid dehydrogenase converts androstenedione to dehydroepiandrosterone
   c. 17α-Hydroxylase is not required to convert deoxycorticosterone to 11-deoxycortisol
   d. 5α-Reductase is required to convert testosterone to dihydrotestosterone
   e. 20,22-Desmolase converts cholesterol to pregnenolone

48. **The following hormonal changes occur during pregnancy**
   a. There is a decrease in unbound cortisol levels
   b. The circulating levels of ACTH decrease during second and third trimesters of pregnancy
   c. TRH causes release of thyroid-stimulating hormone and prolactin
   d. TRH can also cause an increase in ACTH during pregnancy
   e. Prolactin levels rise throughout pregnancy

49. **The cells involved in synthesis of anterior pituitary hormones**
   a. Acidophils secrete prolactin
   b. Acidophils secrete ACTH
   c. Acidophils secrete growth hormone
   d. Basophils secrete gonadotrophins
   e. Basophils secrete TSH

50. **Ovarian wedge resection causes the following hormonal changes**
   a. Increases the serum androgen level
   b. Decreases the intraovarian androgen levels
   c. Increases the available androgen substrate for peripheral aromatization to oestrogen
   d. May decrease the circulating levels of inhibin
   e. Decreases the serum androgen level

51. The complications of laparoscopic ovarian drilling
a. It causes more adhesions compared with ovarian wedge resection (OWR)
b. It may cause ovarian failure in case of excessive electrocoagulation
c. The use of laser is associated with fewer adhesions than electrocautery
d. The use of laser is associated with lower pregnancy rates than electrocautery
e. Adhesions are almost always found after ovarian drilling

52. Severe ovarian hyperstimulation syndrome (OHSS)
a. The pathophysiological hallmark is decreased vascular permeability
b. There is loss of proteins into the third space
c. It can lead to hepatorenal failure
d. It decreases the risk of cerebrovascular thrombosis
e. It increases the risk of deep vein thrombosis

53. Hormones and receptors (site of action)
a. Peptide hormones act predominantly through receptors on the nucleus
b. Steroid hormone usually acts through cell surface receptors
c. FSH is typically linked to the G-protein second messenger system
d. Thyroid hormones act through nuclear receptors
e. Androgens act through intracellular receptors

54. Growth hormone
a. Is a protein with high carbohydrate content
b. Stimulates the synthesis of insulin-like growth factor-I (IGF-I)
c. Is similar to human placental lactogen in its chemical structure
d. Promotes gluconeogenesis
e. Stimulates the synthesis of insulin-like growth factor-II (IGF-II)

55. The secretion of the growth hormone is stimulated by
a. Somatostatin
b. Corticosteroids
c. Hyperglycaemia
d. Arginine
e. Amino acids

56. Testosterone in males promotes development of
a. Seminal vesicles
b. Seminiferous tubules
c. Vas deferens
d. Epididymis
e. Bulk of muscles

57. With regard to synthesis of adrenal hormones

a. Zona reticularis synthesizes oestrogen precursor
b. Zona reticularis synthesizes androgens
c. Zona fasciculata secretes aldosterone
d. ACTH stimulates aldosterone secretion
e. Zona glomerulosa secretes adrenaline

58. Adenocorticotrophic hormone

a. Secretion is controlled by hypothalamus
b. Promotes glucose uptake
c. Mainly promotes cortisol secretion
d. Promotes release of vasopressin
e. Levels normally rise throughout pregnancy

59. The actions of glucocorticoid hormones are

a. Promotes gluconeogenesis in liver
b. Increases potassium reabsorption in the kidneys
c. Causes lymphocytosis in excessive amounts
d. Causes euphoria in excessive amounts
e. Increases sodium reabsorption in the kidneys

60. The following are true with regard to congenital adrenal hyperplasia (CAH)

a. It is an autosomal dominant condition
b. 21-Hydroxylase is the commonest enzyme deficiency seen in CAH
c. It can present in adults as late-onset disease
d. 17-Hydroxyprogesterone is very low in CAH
e. The gene for 21-hydroxylation is located on chromosome 6

61. With respect to testosterone hormone in females

a. Testosterone is predominantly bound to albumin
b. Testosterone is predominantly bound to SHBG
c. Testosterone bound to SHBG is biologically inactive
d. Testosterone bound to albumin is biologically active
e. Testosterone is ten times lower in females than in males

62. Progesterone

a. It promotes potassium excretion
b. It promotes sodium excretion
c. It does not necessarily increase respiratory drive during pregnancy
d. It increases the mitotic activity in the endometrium
e. It is thermogenic

63. Oestrogens
a. Estriol is not bound to SHBG
b. Oestrogen increases the hepatic synthesis of binding proteins
c. Oestrogen stimulates endometrial growth
d. Oestrogen reduces bowel motility
e. Oestrogens inhibit conversion of tryptophan to serotonin

64. With respect to GnRH
a. It is released every 90 minutes during the luteal phase
b. It is released every 90 minutes during the follicular phase
c. It is released in pulses and is not controlled by the pulse generator in the arcuate nucleus
d. It is synthesized in the preoptic area of the hypothalamus
e. It stimulates FSH release

65. The following promote lactation
a. High concentration of oestrogen
b. Fall in progesterone levels
c. Prolactin
d. Dopamine
e. Cabergoline

66. Inhibin
a. Is produced by granulosa cells in the ovary
b. Is produced by theca cells in the ovary
c. Stimulates FSH release
d. Serum levels peak during second trimester of pregnancy
e. Is derived from the fetoplacental unit during pregnancy

67. Human placental lactogen (hPL)
a. Is secreted by cytotrophoblast
b. Promotes glycolysis
c. Promotes lipolysis
d. Reduces glucose utilization
e. Promotes amino acid transfer across placenta

68. Human decidua produce
a. PP14
b. Insulin-like growth factor-binding protein 1
c. Prolactin
d. Oestrogen
e. Testosterone

69. **The corpus luteum produces**
   a. Inhibin A
   b. Inhibin B
   c. Activin
   d. Relaxin
   e. Progesterone

70. **Combined oral contraceptive pills**
   a. Increase blood levels of antithrombin III
   b. Increase the blood levels of FSH by stimulating its secretion
   c. Decrease the blood levels of LH by inhibiting its secretion
   d. Increase the blood levels of iron
   e. Increase the blood levels of copper

71. **Combined oral contraceptive pills increase the risk of**
   a. Deep venous thrombosis
   b. Haemorrhagic strokes in women with hypertension
   c. Hepatocellular adenoma
   d. Prolactinoma of the pituitary gland
   e. Endometriosis

72. **Combined oral contraceptive pill (mechanisms of action)**
   a. It inhibits ovulation
   b. It inhibits oestrogen-mediated positive feedback leading to FSH surge
   c. It increases the receptivity to the blastocyst of the endometrium
   d. It reduces the sperm penetrability of the cervical mucus
   e. It inhibits sperm motility

73. **Combined oral contraceptive pill (usual starting times)**
   a. First day of menstruation
   b. Seventh day after induced early abortion
   c. Tenth day after delivery (non-lactating woman)
   d. One month after molar pregnancy
   e. Tenth day after induced late abortion

74. **Combined oral contraceptive pill (COCP)**
   a. Rarely causes corneal damage in contact lens users
   b. Aggravates glaucoma
   c. Causes obstructive jaundice
   d. Increases the risk of gallstones
   e. Increases the risk of cataract

75. **Pregnant women and changes in serum thyroid hormone levels**
   a. Serum thyroglobulin level is increased
   b. Total T_4 level is increased
   c. Total T_3 level is increased
   d. Free T_4 is unchanged during second trimester
   e. Total T_4 level is decreased

76. Calcitonin
a. Its secretion is stimulated by progesterone
b. Its secretion is inhibited by testosterone
c. Its secretion is stimulated by parathyroid hormone
d. Its levels are controlled by the level of circulating ionized calcium
e. In its absence, plasma calcium levels can be normal

77. Anion gap is increased in the following conditions
a. Alkalosis
b. Ketoacidosis
c. Lactic acidosis
d. Hyperosmolar acidosis
e. Salicylate poisoning

78. Anion gap is increased in overdose of
a. Paraldehyde
b. Bromide
c. Ethylene glycol
d. Paracetamol
e. Salicylate

79. With regard to carbonic acid
a. Its concentration is proportional to PaO_2
b. It readily dissociates to hydrochloric acid
c. Hydrochloric acid and sodium bicarbonate are required for its formation
d. Its concentration in red blood cells is maintained by carbonic anhydrase
e. The hydrogen ions in carbonic acid are derived from hydrochloric acid

80. The following are buffer bases
a. Sodium
b. Phosphate
c. Haemoglobin
d. Plasma proteins
e. Bicarbonate

81. Respiratory alkalosis
a. Is associated with low PCO_2 *and* a low pH
b. Can occur at high altitudes
c. Can be induced by hypoventilation
d. Can be induced by hyperventilation
e. Can occur during panic attacks

82. With regard to alveolar air and ventilation

a. Alveolar air does not contain water
b. Alveolar ventilation is approximately 2 litres for each breath
c. The composition of alveolar gas remains constant
d. Expired air is a mixture of alveolar air and inspired air
e. The alveolar ventilation is approximately 4.2 litres/minute

83. Pregnancy and ventilation

a. Hyperventilation causes a fall in PCO_2
b. Increase in ventilation is much less than increase in O_2 consumption
c. Progesterone decreases the respiratory rate
d. The increase in ventilation is achieved by an increase in the respiratory rate
e. Oestrogen increases the respiratory rate

84. The following are true with regard to gastric emptying

a. Fats are the slowest of all emptying substances
b. Solid food empties before liquids
c. Carbohydrates are the slowest of all emptying substances
d. Hypotonic contents empty before isotonic contents
e. Gastric emptying is inhibited by acid

85. Carotid and aortic body chemoreceptors

a. Carotid body is sensitive to a decrease in PO_2
b. Carotid body is sensitive to the oxygen content in blood
c. Carotid body is sensitive to an increase in PCO_2
d. Aortic body is not sensitive to a decrease in pH
e. Aortic body is sensitive to changes in PCO_2 and pH

86. Glomerular filtration rate

a. Is increased during pregnancy
b. Is directly proportional to body surface area
c. Is 20% more in women than in men
d. Can be measured by radioactive vitamin B_{12} during pregnancy
e. Is normally 120 mL/min

87. With regard to immunoglobulins

a. IgA helps in antigen recognition by cells
b. IgG promotes complement fixation
c. IgE releases histamine from basophils and mast cells
d. IgA protects the epithelial lining of intestines
e. IgD helps in antigen recognition by cells

88. Serum levels of the clotting factors that rise during pregnancy

a. Von Willebrand factor
b. Plasminogen activator inhibitor
c. Tissue plasminogen activator
d. Protein S
e. Fibrinogen

89. **Total iron-binding capacity (TIBC)**
   a. Is increased in iron deficiency anaemia
   b. Is one-third saturated with iron in women without anaemia
   c. Increases in late pregnancy
   d. Decreases in iron deficiency anaemia
   e. Saturation >25% indicates iron deficiency anaemia during pregnancy

90. **Haemochromatosis**
   a. Is due to iron overload in the form of ferritin
   b. Can be acquired or hereditary
   c. In severe form can lead to gonadal atrophy
   d. Can lead to cirrhosis of liver
   e. May present with diabetes

91. **Haemolytic disease of newborn**
   a. Occurs when Rh-negative mother carries Rh-negative fetus
   b. Occurs when Rh-negative mother carries Rh-positive fetus
   c. Occurs when mother is Rh negative and father is Rh negative
   d. Can occur when mother is Rh negative and father is Rh positive
   e. Occurs when mother is Rh positive and father is Rh positive

92. **Physiological changes during pregnancy (blood and blood flow)**
   a. Plasma volume is increased by 50%
   b. Red cell volume is increased by 60%
   c. Blood flow to the kidneys is increased to 400 mL/min
   d. Plasma volume reaches a plateau around 20 weeks
   e. Blood flow to the uterus is increased to 700 mL/min

93. **Blood pressure changes during pregnancy**
   a. Diastolic pressure is reduced in mid-trimester
   b. Systolic pressure changes throughout pregnancy
   c. There is decrease in peripheral vascular resistance
   d. Blood pressure is higher in the supine position than sitting position
   e. Blood pressure is lower in the supine position than sitting position

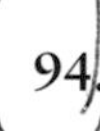

94. **The following are true with regard to suxamethonium**
   a. It is metabolized by serum pseudocholinesterase
   b. It is made of four molecules of acetylcholine
   c. It is used as a muscle relaxant in anaesthesia
   d. It has been used as a muscle relaxant in electroconvulsive therapy
   e. Quick recovery of respiratory paralysis is seen in individuals with abnormal pseudocholinesterase

95. **The following are true regarding fetal circulation**
   a. The blood in the umbilical vein and ductus venosus is 100% saturated with oxygen
   b. Right–left shunt through the foramen ovale is maintained by high venous return from placenta
   c. Right–left shunt through the ductus arteriosus is maintained by high pulmonary vascular resistance
   d. At birth, the ductus arteriosus closes due to direct effect of increasing PCO_2
   e. At birth, the ductus arteriosus closes due to direct effect of increasing PO_2

96. **Hormonal effects on the gastrointestinal system (during pregnancy)**
   a. Gastric emptying time is increased
   b. Lower oesophageal sphincter tone is reduced
   c. The motility of the small intestine is increased
   d. The motility of the large intestine is reduced
   e. The motility of the small intestine is reduced

97. **Heparin**
   a. Is a polysaccharide
   b. Activates the enzyme lipoprotein lipase
   c. Passes through the placenta
   d. Is secreted in the breast milk
   e. Increases the bleeding tendency in a fetus

98. **Narcotic analgesics**
   a. Narcotic analgesics do not cross the placenta
   b. Morphine causes less respiratory depression than tramadol
   c. Codeine is more potent in terms of analgesia than dihydrocodeine
   d. Pentazocine can cause a decrease in blood pressure
   e. Narcotic analgesics can stimulate the chemoreceptor trigger zone

99. **β Agonists**
   a. Promote glycogenolysis
   b. Promote surfactant production
   c. Down-regulate their own receptors
   d. Can cause maternal bradycardia
   e. Promote uterine relaxation

100. **The following are tocolytic agents**
   a. Atosiban oxytocin antagonist)
   b. Entonox
   c. Nifedipine
   d. Magnesium sulphate
   e. Nitroglycerin

101. Mechanism of action of chemotherapeutic drugs
a. Cisplatin – inhibits DNA synthesis
b. Vincristine – interferes with microtubular assembly
c. Actinomycin D – interferes with DNA replication
d. Cyclophosphamide – interferes with RNA replication
e. Vinblastine – binds to tubulin and causes arrest at metaphase

102. The following are matched correctly
a. Cyclophosphamide – haemorrhagic cystitis
b. Melphalan – leukaemia
c. Busulphan – vaginal fibrosis
d. Doxorubicin – supraventricular tachycardia
e. Adriamycin – cardiac toxicity

103. The effects of warfarin on the fetus include
a. Nasal hypoplasia
b. Thymic aplasia
c. Neural tube defects
d. Recurrent intracranial haemorrhage
e. Chondrodysplasia punctata

104. Inhalational anaesthetic agents
a. Etomidate
b. Halothane
c. Ketamine
d. Isoflurane
e. Benzocaine

105. Methyldopa
a. Acts peripherally on α_2-receptors
b. Can cause postural hypotension
c. May cause hepatitis
d. Is teratogenic to fetus
e. Can cause postnatal depression

106. Monoamine oxidase (MAO) inhibitors
a. Reversibly inhibit monoamine oxidase enzyme in the CNS
b. Irreversibly inhibit monoamine oxidase enzyme in the gut
c. Reversibly inhibit monoamine oxidase enzyme in platelets
d. Can cause hypertensive crisis due to increased tyramine absorption
e. Can cause sedation due to antihistaminic properties

107. Antipsychotic drugs
a. Are exclusively excreted via kidneys
b. Are highly lipophilic
c. Can cause tardive dyskinesia
d. Clozepine can cause leucocytosis
e. Chlorprothixene can cause marked extrapyramidal effects

108. **The following are pro-drugs**
a. Cyclophosphamide
b. Cimetidine
c. Levodopa
d. Zidovudine
e. Methyldopa

109. **Drugs that are mainly excreted unchanged in urine include**
a. Digoxin
b. Furosemide
c. Gentamicin
d. Verapamil
e. Methotrexate

110. **Muscarinic drugs acting on postsynaptic acetylcholine receptors include**
a. Atropine
b. Pilocarpine
c. Reserpine
d. Methacholine
e. Bethanechol

111. **Drugs that lower intraocular pressure include**
a. Acetazolamide
b. Bendrofluazide
c. Clonidine
d. Loratadine
e. Timolol

112. **Laxatives and mechanism of action**
a. Lactulose is a mild intestinal stimulant
b. Methycellulose is a bulk-forming agent
c. Liquid paraffin is a bulk-forming agent
d. Dioctyl sodium sulphosuccinate is a faecal softener
e. Castor oil is an osmotic agent

113. **Aprotinin**
a. Is a glycoprotein
b. Is a serine protease inhibitor
c. Potentiates the action of plasmin
d. Potentiates the action of plasminogen
e. Inactivates kallikrein

114. **Low dose aspirin**
a. Reversibly binds to the enzyme cyclooxygenase in platelets
b. Increases the production of thromboxane A_2 in platelets
c. Undergoes first-pass metabolism in kidneys
d. Ingestion within 5 days of delivery is associated with bleeding problems in neonate, e.g. cephalohaematoma
e. Can produce gastric erosion and bleeding

115. Oxytocin causes
a. Bradycardia
b. Hyponatraemia
c. Dehydration
d. Neonatal jaundice
e. Hyperkalaemia

116. Ergometrine
a. Acts within a minute of intravenous injection
b. Acts within a minute of intramuscular injection
c. Causes tonic contraction of the uterus
d. Causes decrease in blood pressure
e. Causes severe vomiting

117. With regard to stillbirths and perinatal deaths
a. Stillbirth is fetal death before 24 weeks of gestation
b. Stillbirth is fetal death after 24 weeks of gestation
c. Stillbirth rate is the number of stillbirths per 1000 live births and stillbirths
d. Perinatal death is stillbirth plus deaths at less than 7 days of life
e. Perinatal death rate is stillbirths plus first week deaths per 1000 live births

118. With regard to neonatal deaths
a. Early neonatal death is death at 0–30 days of life
b. Late neonatal deaths are deaths after 30 days of life
c. Early neonatal death is death at 0–6 days of life
d. Neonatal death rate is the number of deaths at 0–27 days per 1000 live births
e. Postneonatal deaths are deaths at >28 days of life but <1 year

119. Varicella-zoster (VZ) and pregnancy
a. The incidence is 1:2000 during pregnancy
b. Seroprevalence of VZIg in adults is >90%
c. The risk of pneumonia is 50% with primary VZ infection during pregnancy
d. The risk of congenital varicella syndrome is 2% with maternal VZ infection >20 weeks
e. The mortality rate is around 6% with varicella pneumonia during pregnancy

120. Prevalence and incidence
a. Prevalence is a measure of disease occurrence
b. Incidence is a measure of disease occurrence
c. Incidence = prevalence × time
d. Prevalence is total number of cases detected at a particular point of time
e. Incidence is a measure of new cases over a particular period of time

121. The following terms are used to compare numerical data
   a. Mean
   b. Mode
   c. Median
   d. Standard error of mean
   e. Standard deviation

122. The following are correct definitions
   a. Sensitivity is the ability of the test to correctly identify patients who do not have disease
   b. Specificity is the ability of the test to correctly identify patients who have a disease
   c. Positive predictive value (PPV) is the probability of having the condition if the test is positive
   d. Negative predictive value (NPV) is the probability of not having the condition if the test is negative
   e. Prevalence is the probability that the subject has the disease before the test is carried out

123. What are the requirements of the screening test?
   a. The test should have a high sensitivity
   b. The test should have a high specificity
   c. The test should be cost-effective
   d. The test should be safe to apply to the whole population
   e. There should be a latent period in disease progression

124. Relative risk (RR)
   a. Is a measure of association used to interpret cohort study
   b. Is the ratio of the risk in an unexposed group compared with the exposed group
   c. RR = 1 means that there is definite exposure–outcome association
   d. RR of 3 means that there is stronger exposure–outcome association
   e. RR <1 means that the exposure–outcome association is very strong

125. The result of a study of risk factors for caesarean section in obese women showed that spontaneous onset of labour had a relative risk of 0.76 and the use of misoprostol for the induction of labour had a relative risk of 2.8. Which of the following statements are correct with regard to this study?
   a. Spontaneous onset of labour and caesarean section have a very strong association
   b. Spontaneous onset of labour and caesarean section have a moderately strong association
   c. Misoprostol use for induction of labour and caesarean section have a strong association
   d. Misoprostol use for induction of labour is protective and not associated with caesarean section
   e. Spontaneous onset of labour is protective against caesarean section and misoprostol use increases the risk of caesarean section

126. A case–control study
a. Is a prospective longitudinal study
b. Is used to clinically investigate the natural history of disease
c. In such studies, a group of people with disease is compared with a second group without disease
d. In such studies, a large number of patients and controls are required
e. In such studies, recall bias is an important drawback

127. Randomized controlled studies
a. Are observational studies
b. Are the gold standard of clinical research
c. An intervention under investigation is compared with standard treatment
d. An intervention under investigation is compared with a placebo
e. In such studies, patients are allocated in random fashion to the two groups

128. Postpartum haemorrhage (PPH)
a. Is defined as blood loss of >500 mL after caesarean delivery
b. Is more common in multiparous women
c. Atony is the cause in 90% of the cases
d. Trauma is seen in 10% of the cases
e. Coagulation problems occur in around 3% of the cases

129. The following terminologies are correct
a. Preterm birth is delivery before 37 completed weeks of gestation
b. Preterm birth is delivery before 24 completed weeks of gestation
c. Low birth weight is weight <2000 g
d. Very low birth weight is weight <1000 g
e. Extremely low birth weight is weight <500 g

130. The muscles that develop from the first pharyngeal arch are
a. Temporalis
b. Posterior belly of digastric
c. Tensor tympani
d. Stapedius
e. Stylopharyngeus

131. Surfactant
a. Is synthesized by type 1 pneumocytes
b. Reduces the surface tension in the alveoli
c. Increased amounts result in collapse of the lung
d. Lack or inadequate synthesis in preterm babies results in respiratory distress syndrome (RDS)
e. Can be given through an endotracheal tube in newborns

132. With regard to epithelial lining of genital tract in females
  a. Labia majora are lined by squamous epithelium
  b. Labia minora are lined by columnar epithelium
  c. Transformation zone of cervix is lined by squamous epithelium
  d. Fallopian tube is lined by ciliated columnar epithelium
  e. Ovarian surface is lined by cuboidal cells

133. Bacteria
  a. Contain both DNA and RNA
  b. Do not possess a cell wall
  c. Replicate by binary fission
  d. Do not possess mitochondria
  e. Are prokaryotic cells

134. The following are obligate intracellular pathogens
  a. Bacteria
  b. Fungi
  c. Viruses
  d. *Chlamydia*
  e. Rickettsias

135. Endotoxin
  a. Is a protein substance
  b. Is heat labile
  c. Activates macrophages to release interleukins
  d. Can be modified by chemicals to produce a toxoid
  e. Is secreted by bacterial cells

136. The following organisms produce an exotoxin
  a. *Clostridium tetani*
  b. *Clostridium perfringens*
  c. *Clostridium botulinum*
  d. *Corynebacterium diphtheriae*
  e. *Pseudomonas aeruginosa*

137. The following exotoxins are examples of protein synthesis inhibitors
  a. Lipopolysaccharide (LPS)
  b. Diphtheria toxin
  c. Verotoxin
  d. Tetanus toxin
  e. Cholera toxin

138. Obligate anaerobic bacteria include
  a. Mycobacteria
  b. *Pseudomonas* sp.
  c. *Helicobacter* sp.
  d. *Bacteroides* sp.
  e. *Clostridium* sp.

139. *Staphylococcus aureus*
  a. Is a Gram-negative organism
  b. Is a part of normal flora in skin
  c. Produces an endotoxin
  d. Is catalase positive
  e. Can cause toxic shock syndrome

140. *Bacillus anthracis*
  a. Is a Gram-positive spore-forming rod
  b. Is sensitive to ciprofloxacin
  c. Causes woolsorter's disease
  d. Its capsule is made of lipopolysaccharide
  e. Produces exotoxin

141. **Ectoderm gives rise to**
  a. Enamel of teeth
  b. Epidermis
  c. Cartilage
  d. Kidney
  e. Smooth muscle

142. **Functions of skin**
  a. It protects against allergy
  b. It protects against infection
  c. It synthesizes vitamin E
  d. It helps in temperature regulation
  e. It prevents excessive water loss

143. **Herpes simplex virus (HSV)**
  a. Type 1 HSV is spread by direct contact
  b. Type 1 HSV is spread by droplet infection
  c. Type 1 HSV usually affects the genital area
  d. Type 1 HSV can cause painful gingivostomatitis
  e. Type 1 HSV can cause ocular lesions

144. **Molluscum contagiosum**
  a. Is a poxvirus
  b. Is a common skin infection of adulthood
  c. Manifests as small umbilicated lesions on skin (>0.5 cm size)
  d. Exhibits Koebner phenomenon
  e. Always requires treatment

145. **Maternal age-related risk of Down syndrome**
  a. 1:2000 – 20 years
  b. 1:350 – 35 years
  c. 1:240 – 36 years
  d. 1:40 – 40 years
  e. 1:10 – 44 years

146. **Odds ratio (OR)**
   a. Is the measure of the association used to interpret case–control study
   b. Odds ratio = 1 means that there is no difference in outcome in either the exposed or unexposed group
   c. Odds ratio >1 means that the factor under study is a risk factor for outcome
   d. Odds ratio <1 means that the factor under study is a protective factor with respect to outcome
   e. Odds ratio >1 is considered a clinically significant result

147. **Maternal death**
   a. Is death of women while pregnant or within 42 days of termination of pregnancy or from any cause related or aggravated by the pregnancy or its management
   b. Direct deaths are those resulting from previously existing disease leading to death during pregnancy
   c. Indirect deaths are those deaths resulting from conditions that are unique to pregnancy and these may occur during antepartum, intrapartum and postpartum periods
   d. Late deaths are those that occur between 42 days and 1 year of termination of pregnancy, miscarriage or delivery which are due to direct or indirect maternal causes
   e. Coincidental deaths are those that occur during pregnancy due to causes not related to pregnancy

148. **Meta-analysis**
   a. Amalgamation technique to combine statistical results from similar clinical trials
   b. Involves measures to minimize biases of various kinds
   c. Involves measures to minimize the effects of chance
   d. Patients in one trial are directly compared with those in another trial
   e. Summary statistics are calculated for each trial

149. **The following terminologies are correctly matched**
   a. **Placebo treatment** – treatment appears exactly like the comparison treatment but does not contain the active part of the treatment
   b. **Placebo effect** – it results from actual treatment effect rather than the belief that one has been treated
   c. **Single blind** – the subjects being treated do not know which treatment they are receiving
   d. **Double blind** –the subjects being treated and the people evaluating the outcome variables both know which treatment the subjects are receiving
   e. **Hawthorne effect** – a side effect introduced by the act of observation in observational studies

150. In hypothesis testing
a. Null hypothesis specifies a hypothesized real value for a parameter
b. Type I error occurs when the null hypothesis is not rejected when it is false
c. Type II error occurs when the null hypothesis is rejected when it is true
d. The power of the test is the probability of rejecting the null hypothesis when it is false
e. An alternative hypothesis specifies a real value for a parameter which will be considered when the null hypothesis is not rejected

151. Common neonatal pathogens and routes of acquisition
a. HIV – breast milk
b. *S. epidermidis* – central venous catheters
c. Varicella – transplacental
d. Parvovirus – birth canal
e. Herpes simplex virus – birth canal

152. Respiratory distress syndrome (RDS)
a. Is less common in newborn babies born before 34 weeks
b. Is more common in newborn babies born after 36 weeks
c. Antenatal maternal glucocorticoids reduce its incidence in preterm babies
d. Use of surfactant replacement early in newborn preterm babies reduces its incidence
e. Chest radiograph may show ground-glass appearance with air bronchograms

153. Hepatitis E virus
a. Is a double-stranded RNA virus
b. Is a double-stranded DNA virus
c. Belongs to the parvovirus family
d. Is transmitted through blood products
e. Causes chronic liver disease

154. German measles (rubella)
a. Is a chronic infectious disease
b. Is caused by an RNA togavirus
c. Is characterized by a maculopapular rash
d. Is associated with suboccipital lymphadenopathy
e. Koplik spots are pathognomonic for rubella

155. *Rickettsia rickettsii*
a. Is an obligate intracellular bacterium
b. Has a Gram-positive cell envelope
c. Is transmitted by hard ticks
d. Invades the lining of the gastrointestinal tract
e. Causes Rocky Mountain spotted fever

156. **Infectious mononucleosis**
   a. Is common in young children
   b. Is caused by the Epstein–Barr virus (EBV)
   c. Heterophil antibody titre is helpful in diagnosis
   d. It has been associated with Burkitt lymphoma
   e. Aciclovir is used for its treatment

157. **Human papillomavirus (HPV)**
   a. Is a single-stranded DNA virus
   b. It can transfect human keratinocyes
   c. Its genome is made of early and late regions
   d. Early (E) region produces proteins that form its capsid
   e. Late (L) region codes protein responsible for its replication

158. **The following are DNA-containing viruses**
   a. Varicella-zoster
   b. HTLV-1
   c. Cytomegalovirus
   d. Coxsackievirus
   e. Hepatitis B virus

159. ***Treponema pallidum***
   a. Is a spirochaete
   b. Is resistant to drying
   c. Is isolated by culture
   d. Is visualized by dark-ground illumination under microscopy
   e. Crosses the placenta before 16 weeks of pregnancy

160. ***Mycobacterium tuberculosis***
   a. Is less resistant to drying
   b. Ziehl–Neelsen method is used for staining
   c. Resists decolorization by alcohol after staining
   d. Takes 1 week to grow in culture
   e. Löwenstein–Jensen medium is used for its culture

161. **Human immunodeficiency virus (HIV)**
   a. Contains reverse transcriptase
   b. Contains both DNA and RNA
   c. Can synthesize DNA from its RNA
   d. Gains entry into T-helper cells
   e. Can be transmitted by artificial insemination

162. ***Neisseria gonorrhoeae***
   a. Is a Gram-positive diplococcus
   b. Is sensitive to cold
   c. Needs 5% oxygen to grow
   d. Needs Stuart medium for its transport
   e. Monoarticular arthritis is an early complication

163. Lyme disease
- a. Is caused by *Borrelia burgdorferi*
- b. Is transmitted by mouse bites
- c. Is associated with the rash – erythema chronicum migrans
- d. Is associated with granuloma formation
- e. Can be associated with fever and lymphadenopathy

164. Parvovirus B19
- a. Causes erythema infectiosum
- b. Can cause arthralgia in adults
- c. Causes aplastic anaemia in fetus
- d. Is a recognized cause of hydrops in fetus
- e. Presents with characteristic facial rash in children

165. *Mycobacterium leprae*
- a. Is an acid-fast bacillus
- b. Does not cause granuloma formation
- c. Has a predilection for the cutaneous nerves
- d. Has a predilection for the liver
- e. Gram stain is used for staining

166. Hepatitis B virus
- a. Belongs to herpes viruses
- b. Its genome is made of DNA
- c. Its nucleocapsid encloses DNA polymerase
- d. Its nucleocapsid core is made of lipid
- e. Uses reverse transcription for its replication

167. *Trichomonas vaginalis*
- a. Is a sexually transmitted infection
- b. Is a single-celled bacterium
- c. It may survive up to 45 minutes outside the body
- d. Trichomoniasis is associated with decreased risk of HIV transmission
- e. Is transmitted through oral sex

168. Bacterial vaginosis
- a. Causes an increase in the vaginal pH
- b. Is caused only by pathogen *Gardnerella vaginalis*
- c. Is associated with a characteristic fishy odour
- d. Is associated with an increase in lactobacilli in the vagina
- e. The whiff test is positive

169. *Chlamydia trachomatis*
- a. Is a facultative intracellular bacterium
- b. Is causative organism for lymphogranuloma venereum
- c. Is the commonest cause of non-gonococcal urethritis in men
- d. Is the most common cause of PID in women
- e. Can cause pneumonia in neonate

170. **Methyldopa**
   a. Is a central α_2-receptor agonist
   b. Is metabolized in the kidneys
   c. Is excreted in urine
   d. Can cause lupus erythematosus-like syndrome
   e. Is used as first-line antihypertensive agent in pregnant women

171. **Gap junctions in myometrium**
   a. Decrease in number prior to labour
   b. Numbers are regulated by oestrogen
   c. Numbers are regulated by prostaglandins
   d. Asynchronize the myometrial function during labour
   e. Smooth muscle cells communicate via these junctions

172. **During labour oestrogen causes**
   a. A decrease in cAMP levels via α-adrenergic receptors
   b. A decrease in the number of oxytocin receptors
   c. An increase in production of $PGF_{2\alpha}$
   d. A decrease in the myometrial gap junctions
   e. An increase in cAMP via β-adrenergic receptors

173. **With regard to prostaglandins during pregnancy and labour**
   a. Induces uterine contractions only in first trimester when administered
   b. PGE_2 and $PGF_{2\alpha}$ are both produced in human decidua
   c. $PGF_{2\alpha}$ is exclusively produced in human chorion and amnion
   d. Causes cervical ripening or softening of the cervix during labour
   e. $PGF_{2\alpha}$ and PGE_2 relax the cervical smooth muscle

174. **The following are contraindications to β-agonist tocolytic therapy during pregnancy**
   a. Thyrotoxicosis
   b. Uncontrolled diabetes
   c. Mild asthma
   d. History of epilepsy
   e. Severe cardiac disease

175. **β-Adrenergic receptor agonists**
   a. Promote surfactant production in fetal lungs
   b. Decrease uterine blood flow causing myometrial contraction
   c. Similar to oxytocin, down-regulate their own receptors in the myometrium
   d. May have direct stimulant effect on the fetal heart
   e. Can be used with monoamine oxidase inhibitors

1. Practice MCQs 1: Answers

1a. True
1b. True
1c. False
1d. True
1e. False

Note
The pelvic brim is the superior opening of the pelvis or pelvic inlet. It is bounded by the sacral promontory (behind), the iliopectineal line (the ridge going over the ilium and pectin pubis) defining the lateral aspect of the pelvic brim, and is bounded by pubis symphysis anteriorly. The following structures pass over the pelvic brim: superior rectal artery, gonadal arteries, ureters and psoas muscle.

2a. False
2b. True
2c. False
2d. True
2e. False

Note
Urogenital diaphragm – the sheath of muscle enclosed between the two triangular fascial membranes. The superior layer is thin and the inferior layer is tough and fibrous. It lies inferior to the pelvic diaphragm. Posteriorly, it encloses the deep transverse perineal muscle and anteriorly, it encloses the urethral sphincter.

3a. True
3b. True
3c. False
3d. False
3e. False

Note
Ischiorectal fossa – these are triangular spaces, which contain fat. The apex is formed by the levator ani muscle, laterally bounded by the obturator internus muscle, the anal canal forms the medial aspect, the posterior aspect is bounded by the gluteus maximus muscle and sacrotuberous ligament, and perineal skin forms the base.

4a. False
4b. False
4c. False
4d. True
4e. True

Note

The pudendal canal contains the pudendal artery, pudendal vein and pudendal nerve. It runs in the lateral wall of the ischiorectal fossa and medial to the obturator internus muscle. It travels out through the greater sciatic foramen and is in close association with ischial spines (lateral to ischial spines). It travels back through the lesser sciatic foramen and runs along the medial aspect of the ischiopubic ramus.

5a. False
5b. True
5c. False
5d. True
5e. False

Note

Course of ureter in the abdomen and pelvis

The abdominal part lies on the psoas major and anteriorly crosses the genitofemoral nerve. It then enters the pelvis (passes the pelvic brim along the posterior wall) in front of the common iliac or external iliac vessels. It follows the anterior border of the greater sciatic notch and turns medially at the ischial spines. It then runs in the base of the broad ligament before it reaches the bladder. In the broad ligament (mainly parametrium) the uterine artery crosses the ureter superiorly (often termed 'water under the bridge') before entering the uterus. The ureter then runs above the lateral fornix of the vagina (2 cm lateral to the cervix) and turns medially in front of the vagina to enter the bladder. It is retroperitoneal in most of its course except towards the ending before entering the bladder. The nerve supply comes from the sympathetic nerves (T11 to L1).

6a. True
6b. False
6c. True
6d. False
6e. True

Note

Ovaries are located in the ovarian fossa (the anterior boundary is the obliterated umbilical artery and the posterior boundary is the ureter and internal iliac artery). The ovaries are held in position by the ovarian ligament and suspensory ligament.

The surface of the ovary is lined by cuboidal cells (germinal epithelium) and beneath this is tunica albuginea. The ovary has a cortex (contains follicles and corpora lutea) and vascular medulla. The ovum is released into the peritoneal cavity at mid-cycle and is picked up by the fimbrial end of the fallopian tube.

The major blood vessels enter the ovary at the ovarian hilum. Both ovarian arteries arise from the abdominal aorta. The left ovarian vein drains into left renal and right ovarian vein drains into inferior vena cava. The lymphatics of the ovary drain into the para-aortic nodes. The parasympathetic nerve supply comes from the vagus nerve and the sympathetic nerve supply comes from T10 (lesser splanchnics, via the hypogastric to the ovarian plexus).

7a. False
7b. False
7c. True
7d. True
7e. True

Note

The pelvic bone is divided into different parts (ilium, ischium and pubic bone). The ilium consists of iliac crest, lateral surface, medial surface (pelvic surface or iliac fossa), iliac tuberosity, anteroinferior iliac spines and anterosuperior iliac spine.

The iliac crest is the superior portion of the iliac bone and the most prominent part of the ilium. The iliac tubercles are bony prominences on the iliac crest. The antero- and posterosuperior iliac spines are the projections at each end of the iliac crest. The muscles attached to the iliac crest are external oblique muscle, internal oblique muscle, latissimus dorsi, transversus abdominis and quadratus lumborum.

Gluteal muscles are attached to the lateral surface of the ilium and iliacus is attached to the medial surface. Inguinal ligament and sartorius muscle are attached to the anterosuperior iliac spine and rectus femoris is attached to the anteroinferior iliac spine. The sacroiliac ligament and erector spinae muscle are attached to the iliac tuberosity.

8a. True
8b. False
8c. True
8d. True
8e. False

Note

The internal iliac artery divides into anterior and posterior trunks. The anterior trunk gives rise to visceral braches and parietal branches. The visceral branches are the superior vesical artery (supplies lower ureter and upper bladder), the inferior vesical artery (supplies bladder base and ureter), and the middle rectal, uterine and vaginal arteries. The parietal branches are the obturator, internal pudendal and inferior gluteal arteries.

The posterior trunk of the internal iliac artery gives rise to the superior gluteal, lateral sacral and iliolumbar arteries. The obturator artery runs with its vein below and nerve above in the obturator canal. The anastomosis between the obturator artery and the pubic branch of the inferior epigastric artery is very important, as sometimes this may be a large vessel running lateral or medial to the femoral canal.

9a. True
9b. True
9c. True
9d. False
9e. False – Drain into external iliac nodes.

Note

The lymphatic drainage of the pelvis forms plexus in the individual organs and usually follows the line of the blood vessels. Lymphatics from the uterus mainly drain into external iliac nodes and internal iliac nodes. A few branches along the round ligament drain into superficial inguinal nodes. The cervix mainly drains to the internal iliac nodes and also sometimes to the obturator and external iliac nodes. The upper third of the vagina drains into external iliac nodes, middle third to the internal iliac nodes and lower third to the inguinal nodes. The ovaries drain to para-aortic nodes.

10a. False – suspensory ligament of ovary – it connects the ovary to the lateral pelvic wall.
10b. True
10c. False – round ligament – it runs from the fundus of the uterus to the labia majora (inferolaterally).
10d. False – ovarian ligament – it connects the ovary to the uterus.
10e. True

11a. True
11b. False – it passes the pelvic brim, along the posterior wall. It starts at T12 and passes all along the vertebral column before it enters the pelvis.
11c. True
11d. True
11e. False – it is innervated by L2–4.

12a. True
12b. False
12c. True
12d. True
12e. True

Note

The course of the abdominal aorta, its relations and branches

The aorta enters the abdomen (through the aortic hiatus) behind the diaphragm in between the crura (left and right crus of the diaphragm), at the level of T12. It runs slightly towards the left in front of the first four lumbar vertebrae and ends at the level of L4 where it bifurcates into the left and right common iliac arteries. The inferior vena cava lies to the right and passes behind the aorta at bifurcation. The left renal vein crosses in front of the aorta. The aorta passes posterior to the horizontal portion of the duodenum (third part), the uncinate process and the body of pancreas.

The main branches of the abdominal aorta are the coeliac trunk, superior mesenteric artery, inferior mesenteric artery, renal artery and ovarian artery.

The anterior branches are the coeliac trunk, superior mesenteric and inferior mesenteric arteries. The posterior branches are the lumbar and median sacral arteries. The lateral branches are the inferior phrenic arteries, and renal, ovarian and middle suprarenal arteries.

13a. False
13b. True
13c. False
13d. False
13e. True

Note
Popliteal fossa
It is a diamond-shaped fossa located behind the knee. Superolaterally it is bounded by biceps femoris, superomedially by semimembranosus and semitendinosus and inferiorly by the lateral and medial heads of gastrocnemius. The floor is formed by the popliteal surface of the femur, knee joint capsule and popliteal muscle (superior to inferior).

It contains the popliteal artery, popliteal vein and tibial nerve. The popliteal artery arises here whereas the popliteal vein ends. The order of relation of the above structures from medial to lateral is artery, vein and tibial nerve.

Applied anatomy
The popliteal artery is the deepest structure and lies close to the femur. Thus it can be injured by a fracture of the supracondylar region of the femur.

14a. True
14b. True
14c. False
14d. True
14e. False

Note
Content of the urogenital triangle and attachment of perineal muscles
It contains openings of the vagina plus urethra and crura of the clitoris. The ischiocavernosus muscles arise from the medial aspect of the ischial ramus and enclose the crura of the clitoris.

The bulb of the vestibule is surrounded by the bulbocavernosus muscle, which arises from the perineal body and inserts into the body of the clitoris. It interdigitates with the external anal sphincter before its insertion.

The superficial and deep transverse perineal muscles arise from the perineal body and insert into the ischial ramus. Bartholin's gland and the urogenital diaphragm also lie in the urogenital triangle.

15a. True
15b. True
15c. True

15d. True
15e. False

Note
In females, the round ligament and the ilioinguinal nerve pass through the inguinal canal. In males, the spermatic cord (the contents of the spermatic cord are the testicular artery, pampiniform venous plexus, spermatic fasciae, vas deferens and testicular artery) and ilioinguinal nerve pass through the inguinal canal.

16a. False
16b. False
16c. True
16d. False
16e. True

Note
The inguinal canal has a roof, floor and anterior and posterior walls. The roof is formed by internal oblique and transversus abdominis muscles. The floor is formed by inguinal ligament. The anterior wall is formed by the aponeurosis of the external + internal oblique muscles. The posterior wall is formed by transverse fascia (weak area) and the conjoint tendon (which reinforces the medial part). The aponeurosis of internal oblique and transversus abdominis muscle forms the conjoint tendon.

17a. False
17b. True
17c. True
17d. False
17e. False

Note
The nerves supplying the lower limbs include the femoral, obturator, tibial, common peroneal, superficial peroneal and deep peroneal nerves. The femoral nerve supplies the anterior compartment of the thigh – sartorius, quadriceps femoris and pectineus. The obturator nerve supplies the medial compartment of the thigh – adductor longus and brevis, gracilis, anterior portion of adductor magnus. The tibial nerve supplies the posterior compartment of the thigh (semimembranosus, semitendinosus, long head of biceps femoris and posterior portion of adductor magnus) and the posterior compartment of the leg (gastrocnemius, soleus, flexor digitorum longus, flexor hallucis longus and tibialis posterior). It also supplies plantar muscles of the foot.

The common peroneal nerve supplies the short head of biceps femoris. It divides into superficial and deep peroneal branches, which supply the muscles of the leg. The anterior compartment is supplied by deep peroneal nerve, the posterior compartment by tibial nerve and the lateral compartment by superficial peroneal nerve. The deep peroneal nerve supplies tibialis anterior, extensor digitorum, extensor hallucis and peroneus tertius. The superficial peroneal nerve supplies peroneus longus and brevis.

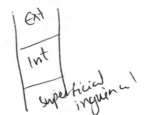

18a. False
18b. True
18c. False
18d. False
18e. True

Note
The anterior rami of spinal nerves (T12 to S4) form the lumbosacral plexus. The innervation of the lower limb is derived from segments L2 to S3. The femoral nerve is derived from L2 to L4 (posterior division). The tibial nerve is derived from L4 to S3 (anterior division). The obturator nerve is derived from L2 to L4 (anterior division). The common peroneal nerve is derived from L4 to S2 (posterior division).

19a. True
19b. False – the middle third drains into the internal iliac nodes.
19c. False – the upper third generally drains into the external iliac nodes.
19d. True – posterior vagina drains into inferior gluteal, sacral and anorectal nodes, ultimately draining into internal iliac nodes.
19e. False

20a. True
20b. True
20c. True
20d. True
20e. True

Note
Trisomy 18 is also called Edwards syndrome. The incidence is 1:5000 newborns. Fetal loss (85%) usually occurs between 10 weeks and term and those born alive die in 2 months (<10% survive to 1 year). In addition to the features described, it is associated with abnormalities of the skeletal system, omphalocele, intrauterine growth retardation and severe learning disability.

21a. False
21b. True
21c. False
21d. True
21e. True

Note
The regions on the chromosome that are vulnerable to separate or break under certain manipulations are called the fragile site. The fragile site on the long arm of the X chromosome (Xq27) has been correlated with the altered phenotype and is called fragile X syndrome.

It is more common in males than females and the incidence in males is 1:1000 while in females it is 1:2000. It is characterized by learning disability, large ears, large testes and a prominent jaw. While considering the cause for learning disability due to chromosomal abnormalities, fragile X syndrome stands second to Down syndrome.

22a. True
22b. True
22c. True
22d. False
22e. True

Note
Non-dysjunction in the male gamete is the cause in 80% of these women. The remainder are either due to structural abnormalities of the X chromosome or mitotic non-dysjunction resulting in mosaicism. It is characterized by short stature, webbed neck, broad chest with wide-spaced nipples, lymphoedema of the extremities and heart defects.

23a. True
23b. True
23c. True
23d. True
23e. True

Note
Abnormalities in chromosome number can occur during mitosis or meiosis. During meiosis, two members of a pair of homologous chromosomes normally separate at the first meiotic division and this results in each daughter cell receiving one member of each pair. If separation does not occur, both members of a pair will move into one cell. This is called non-dysjunction.

For example, if one cell receives 24 chromosomes and the other 22 (normal 23). If a gamete having 23 chromosomes fuses with a gamete of 24 chromosomes, the result is 47 chromosomes (trisomy). This can happen during the first or second meiotic division.

24a. True
24b. False
24c. True
24d. False
24e. True

Note
Down syndrome is trisomy 21. The features of Down syndrome in children include flat facies, small ears, cardiac abnormalities, epicanthic folds, craniofacial abnormalities, upward slanting eyes, hypotonia, and growth retardation and learning disability. There is a high incidence of leukaemia, infection, thyroid dysfunction and premature ageing in these individuals.

Ninety-five per cent of the cases are due to meiotic non-dysjunction.

Four per cent of the cases are due to unbalanced translocation between chromosome 21 and chromosome 13, 14 or 15.

Only 1% is due to mosaicism resulting from mitotic non-dysjunction. They may not have all the features of Down syndrome.

25a. True
25b. False
25c. True
25d. True
25e. True

Note
The changes that take place in the transformation of spermatids into spermatozoa are called spermatogenesis.

Spermatogenesis is regulated by the hormone LH. This binds to receptors in the Leydig cells and promotes testosterone production, which in turn binds to Sertoli cells to promote spermatogenesis. Sertoli cells stimulate secretion of intracellular androgen receptor proteins.

The time required for a spermatogonium to develop into a mature spermatozoon is around 64 days. Spermatozoa enter the lumen of seminiferous tubules once fully formed. Thereafter they are pushed towards the epididymis and obtain full motility in the epididymis.

26a. True
26b. False – cranial neuropore closing or closed.
26c. False – caudal neuropore closing or closed.
26d. True
26e. True – caudal neuropore also open.

27a. True
27b. False – by 12 weeks of fetal development, primary ossification centre develops in the skull.
27c. False – only primary ossification centres develop in the long bones.
27d. True – the umbilical herniation occurs at the sixth week and the intestinal loops are floating in the extra-embryonic coelomic cavity. They are withdrawn into the abdominal cavity by 12 weeks.
27e. True – the external genitalia are well developed by 12 weeks and therefore sex can be determined by ultrasound.

Note
The point in the cartilage where ossification starts is termed the ossification centre. The primary ossification centres usually appear during the prenatal developmental period and are in the diaphysis of the long bones, while most secondary ossification centres appear during the postnatal and adolescent period and are located in the epiphysis of the long bones.

28a. True
28b. False – it is replaced every 3 hours.
28c. True – it acts as a protective cushion to the fetus.
28d. True – the fetus starts swallowing amniotic fluid by the beginning of the fifth month and also adds to amniotic fluid by its contribution as urine.
28e. True

Note
Amniotic fluid (clear, watery fluid) is produced by amniocytes and the main contribution is from the maternal circulation (blood). It is 30 mL at 10 weeks, 450 mL at 20 weeks and 800–1000 mL at 37 weeks.

29a. True – it is also failure of the herniated bowel to come back to the abdominal cavity (this is physiological between 6 and 10 weeks).
29b. False – it is associated with severe malformations (cardiac defects in 50% and neural tube defects in 40%).
29c. True – it can also contain bladder and small and large intestine.
29d. False – it is associated with a high mortality rate (25%).
29e. True

Note
The incidence of omphalocele is 2.5/10 000 births while gastroschisis is 1/10 000 births. Gastroschisis is herniation of the bowel through the abdominal wall into the amniotic cavity and the defect is lateral to the umbilicus (usually right side). It is not usually associated with chromosomal abnormalities, unlike omphalocele, and consequently survival is good.

30a. True
30b. True
30c. True
30d. True
30e. False

Note
All the above syndromes are associated with skeletal defects. Craniosynostosis occurs in 1:2500 births and is seen in various genetic syndromes. Craniosynostosis is premature closure of one or more sutures of the skull. The closure of different suture lines leads to different shapes of the skull. For example, premature closure of the coronal suture results in a short and high skull and is known as acrocephaly, whereas premature closure of the sagittal suture results in a long and narrow skull and is known as scaphocephaly.

31a. True
31b. False
31c. True
31d. True
31e. True

Note
The metanephros arises at the fifth week and gives rise to the permanent kidney. Its excretory units develop from metanephric mesoderm. The collecting ducts of the kidney develop from the ureteric bud. This is an outgrowth of the mesonephric duct before it enters the cloaca.

32a. False
32b. True
32c. True
32d. False
32e. False

Note
There are two mesonephric ducts (wolffian duct system) and two paramesonephric duct (müllerian duct system) in the body during embryonic development of the reproductive organs. The paramesonephric duct arises from the invagination of the epithellum covering the urogenital ridge on the anterolateral surface. It opens cranially into the abdominal cavity. Caudally, it lies lateral to the mesonephric duct before crossing it ventrally. It then lies medial to the mesonephric duct. Further to this, it joins the opposite paramesonephric duct in the midline and forms the uterine cavity.

In females, the paramesonephric duct gives rise to the uterus, fallopian tubes, cervix, upper third of the vagina (lower two-thirds of the vagina develop from urogenital sinus) and a vestigial or rudimentary structure called Morgagni hydatid. In males, it forms the vestigial structure called the appendix of testis.

33a. True
33b. True
33c. False
33d. True
33e. False – the gubernaculum forms the round ligament.

Note
In males, the mesonephric system (wolffian system) gives rise to structures such as the epididymis, ductus deferens, seminal vesicles, ejaculatory duct, and vestigial or rudimentary structures called paradidymis and appendix of epididymis.

34a. False – mons pubis arises from genital swellings.
34b. True – in males, genital fold gives rise to ventral aspect of the penis.
34c. True – in males, genital swellings give rise to scrotum.
34d. True
34e. False – clitoris arises from the genital tubercle.

35a. False
35b. False
35c. False
35d. True
35e. True

Note
This is also known as testicular feminization syndrome. It is an X-linked recessive disorder. The incidence is 1:20 000 live births. The chromosome is 46XY. The external appearance is female (normal breast development but absent pubic and axillary hair) and the internal organs are male (testes). The uterus and tubes are absent. The vagina is short and blind. The syndrome is a

result of either lack of androgen receptors or failure of the tissues to respond to androgen-receptor complexes (dihydrotestosterone). Although androgens are produced by testes, male differentiation of the genitalia does not occur due to the above reasons.

The testis is generally found in the inguinal region and spermatogenesis does not occur but will produce androgens. These testes are at high risk of developing cancer, with approximately 33% developing a malignancy before the age of 50 years.

36a. True
36b. True
36c. True
36d. True
36e. True

Note
Some cells from the lateral border of the neuroectoderm are separated when the neural folds fuse. These cells form the neural crest and give rise to various structures or tissues. The cells undergo functional (epithelial to mesenchymal) differentiation and travel in different regions to give rise to various specialized tissues.

In the trunk region, the cells leave the neural crest (after closure of the neural tube) and either migrate dorsally through the dermis to form melanocytes or ventrally through the anterior half of somites to become sensory ganglia, sympathetic neurons, enteric neurons, Schwann cells and cells of adrenal medulla.

Neural crest cells that leave the cranial neural folds do so before the closure of the neural tube in this region. These cells give rise to neurons for cranial ganglia, glial cells, melanocytes and craniofascial skeleton.

The other structures that arise from the neural crest are C cells of the thyroid gland, connective tissue and bones of the face and skull, parasympathetic ganglia of the GI tract, dorsal root ganglia of the spinal cord, sympathetic chain and pre-aortic ganglia, and dermis in the face and neck.

37a. True
37b. True
37c. False
37d. True
37e. True

Note
The placental exchange takes place in those villi where the fetal vessels are in intimate contact with syncytiotrophoblastic cells.

During the first trimester the villi are large. The placental membrane consists of four layers: endothelial lining of fetal vessels, mesenchymal tissue in villous core, cytotrophoblast and syncytiotrophoblast.

At this stage, the fetal vessels are small and centrally placed in the loose mesenchymal tissue of villous stroma. These changes are seen in the first trimester and more evident towards the end of the first trimester.

From the fourth month onwards, further changes occur: the villi get smaller and cytotrophoblastic cells appear to be less numerous and fetal vessels are larger in diameter and starting to move towards the periphery of the villus.

From the seventh month onwards, the villi are much smaller in diameter with very few cytotrophoblastic cells. The syncytiotrophoblastic cells are much thinner and anuclear in most areas, and mainly help in gaseous transfer. The fetal vessels in the villi are sinusoidally dilated and occupy most of the cross-sectional area in the villus and take a subtrophoblastic position.

The above changes occur to optimize the maternofetal transfer of nutrients and effective gaseous exchange.

38a. True
38b. True
38c. True
38d. False
38e. True

Note
α-Fetoprotein (AFP) is produced by fetal liver and peaks at around 14 weeks. Maternal serum levels increase during the second trimester and start to steadily decline after 30 weeks of pregnancy.

It is increased in maternal serum and in amniotic fluid in various conditions, e.g. sacrococcygeal teratoma, duodenal atresia, bladder exstrophy, spina bifida, anencephaly, gastroschisis and omphalocele.

AFP levels are decreased in conditions such as Down syndrome (trisomy 21), triploidy and Edwards syndrome (trisomy 18).

These changes form the basis of it being one of the parameters in the quadruple test for Down syndrome, the others being βhCG, estriol and inhibin.

39a. True
39b. False – prolactin is evolutionarily related to growth hormone.
39c. False – prolactin is structurally related to growth hormone.
39d. True
39e. True

40a. True
40b. True
40c. False – dopamine inhibits prolactin secretion.
40d. True
40e. True

Note
Thyrotrophin-releasing hormone (TRH) also promotes prolactin secretion.

41a. False – bulimia nervosa is an eating disorder and does not give rise to raised prolactin.
41b. True
41c. False – anorexia nervosa does not cause hyperprolactinaemia.
41d. True
41e. False

Note
The physiological causes of raised prolactin include pregnancy, lactation, breast stimulation, stress, sexual intercourse and exercise.

The pathological causes of increase in prolactin levels are pituitary adenomas (micro- and macroprolactinomas), PCOS, chronic renal failure, herpes zoster pain, drugs (phenothiazines, haloperidol, metoclopramide, methyldopa, morphine, methadone, oestrogens, cocaine and cimetidine).

42a. False – it is a dopamine agonist and is used in the treatment of hyperprolactinaemia.
42b. True
42c. False – it is a dopamine agonist and is used in the treatment of hyperprolactinaemia.
42d. True
42e. False – it is a dopamine agonist and is used in the treatment of hyperprolactinaemia.

Note
The drugs causing hyperprolactinaemia are not used in the treatment of hyperprolactinaemia, e.g. phenothiazines, haloperidol, metoclopramide, methyldopa, morphine, methadone, oestrogens, cocaine and cimetidine.

43a. False
43b. True
43c. False – promotes prolactin secretion.
43d. True
43e. True

Note
Oxytocin is produced in the supraoptic and paraventricular nuclei of the hypothalamus but is stored and released by the posterior pituitary. It promotes prolactin secretion and also uterine prostaglandin release.

44a. True – in females, usually breast growth and growth spurt occur first. This is followed by the appearance of axillary hair and then menstruation.
44b. False – breast development occurs in five stages.
44c. True
44d. False – the growth spurt usually starts 12 months after increase in the testicular volume in boys.
44e. True

45a. True
45b. True
45c. False – two-thirds of the daily female testosterone production is of ovarian origin.
45d. False – androgens are mainly excreted as 17-oxosteroids after metabolism.
45e. True

46a. False – the half-life of the LH is 20 minutes.
46b. True
46c. True
46d. True
46e. True

Note
The gonadotrophins are metabolized in the liver and kidneys. The half-life of LH is 20 minutes. FSH and LH levels are high during menstruation and tend to fall during the luteal phase of the cycle. Oestrogen exerts both positive and negative feedback (mediated mainly through the pituitary). Frequent pulses of GnRH cause diminished gonadotrophin response (mainly seen in early puberty).

47a. False
47b. False
47c. False
47d. True
47e. True

Note
Synthesis of steroid hormones requires various enzymes. The above are a few examples and one needs to be thorough with the cycle of hormone synthesis to answer the above questions.

48a. False – ACTH levels increase during pregnancy and so do the total and unbound cortisol levels.
48b. False
48c. True
48d. True
48e. True

49a. True
49b. False – basophils produce ACTH.
49c. True
49d. True
49e. True

Note
The anterior pituitary consists of three types of cells. (a) Chromophobes – normally do not secrete any hormone and are called resting cells.
(b) Acidophils – secrete prolactin and growth hormone. (c) Basophils – secrete TSH, ACTH and gonadotrophins. The paraventricular and supraoptic

nuclei synthesize oxytocin and vasopressin. The axons of these nuclei pass on to the posterior pituitary.

50a. False – decreases the serum androgen level.
50b. True
50c. False – decreases the available androgen substrate.
50d. True
50e. True

51a. False – it causes fewer adhesions than ovarian wedge resection.
51b. True
51c. False – it is associated with more adhesions than electrocautery.
51d. True
51e. False

52a. False – it causes increased vascular permeability.
52b. True
52c. True
52d. False – it increases the risk of thrombosis.
52e. True

Note
Severe OHSS is a life-threatening emergency condition. It causes contraction of the intravascular volume, expansion of the third space (ascites, pericardial effusions), severe haemoconcentration and the development of hepatorenal failure. These patients are at risk of developing intravascular thrombosis (DVT, PE or cerebrovascular thrombosis). Cerebrovascular thrombosis, renal failure and cardiac tamponade have been reported as causes of death in women with severe OHSS.

53a. False – peptides act through cell surface receptors.
53b. False – steroid hormones usually act through intracellular receptors.
53c. True
53d. True
53e. True

Note
Hormones can act at various sites. The free hormone is usually the active fraction of the hormone that is available to bind to specific receptors on the cells for inducing effects. The other hormones linked to the G protein second messenger system are LH and TSH. Steroid hormones, vitamin D, retinoic acid and thyroid hormones act through nuclear receptors.

54a. False – growth hormone is a protein with molecular weight of 21 500 Da, and does not contain carbohydrate.
54b. True
54c. True

54d. False – it promotes lipolysis and antagonizes insulin action.
54e. True

Note
Growth hormone is a protein with a molecular weight of 21 500 Da and does not contain carbohydrate. Its effect is mediated through IGF-1. The structure is similar to prolactin and human placental lactogen. It is secreted in short bursts and levels are high in the first part of the night. Growth hormone is stimulated by amino acids, hypoglycaemia and stress. Its secretion is inhibited by glucose.

55a. False – growth hormone is stimulated by amino acids and stress.
55b. False
55c. False – growth hormone secretion is stimulated by hypoglycaemia.
55d. True
55e. True

56a. True
56b. False – testosterone is responsible for development of a wolffian duct in males.
56c. True
56d. True
56e. True

Note
Luteinizing hormone regulates spermatogenesis. It binds to the receptors on Leydig cells and stimulates production of testosterone, which in turn promotes spermatogenesis by binding to Sertoli cells.

57a. True
57b. True
57c. False
57d. False
57e. False

Note
The adrenal gland is divided into the outer cortex and inner medulla. The cortex is further divided into three zones. (a) Outer, zona glomerulosa – secretes mineralocorticoids (aldosterone). (b) Middle, zona fasciculata – primarily secretes glucocorticoids, e.g. cortisol. (c) Inner, zona reticularis – secretes small quantities of androgens. The outer zone is under the control of the renin–angiotensin system and the middle/inner zones are under the control of ACTH.

Mnemonic
G – zona glomerulosa – mineralocorticoids.
F – zona fasciculata – glucocorticoids.
R – zona reticularis – androgens.

58a. True
58b. True
58c. True
58d. False – vasopressin promotes ACTH release.
58e. True

59a. True
59b. False – promotes sodium reabsorption.
59c. False – it causes lymphopenia.
59d. True
59e. True

60a. False – it is autosomal recessive.
60b. True
60c. True
60d. False – 17-hydroxyprogesterone levels are very high in CAH and this is one of the investigations performed for its diagnosis.
60e. True

61a. False – it is predominantly bound to SHBG.
61b. True
61c. True
61d. True
61e. True

Note
85% of testosterone is bound to SHBG and is metabolically inactive; 10–15% is bound to albumin and 1–2% is free. Free and albumin-bound testosterone are biologically active.

62a. False – progesterone promotes sodium excretion.
62b. True
62c. False – it increases respiratory drive during pregnancy.
62d. False – it decreases the mitotic activity.
62e. True

63a. True
63b. True
63c. True
63d. True
63e. True

Note
Both oestrogens and progesterones are produced by the ovary. Oestrogen stimulates endometrial growth and uterine growth. Both oestrogen and progesterone reduce bowel motility. Progesterone increases the respiratory drive and the body temperature and promotes sodium secretion.

64a. True
64b. False
64c. False
64d. True
64e. True

Note
The pituitary is regulated by various hormones such as GnRH, TRH and CRH. GnRH stimulates LH and FSH. It is released in pulses and varies with the menstrual cycle. During the follicular phase, GnRH is released every 60 minutes and during the luteal phase every 90 minutes. It is composed of 10 amino acids and is synthesized in the preoptic area.

65a. False – breast growth during pregnancy is promoted by oestrogens, progesterones, human placental lactogen and prolactin.
65b. True
65c. True
65d. False – dopamine inhibits prolactin secretion.
65e. False – cabergoline (dopamine agonist) inhibits prolactin secretion and therefore inhibits lactation.

Note
The lactogenic effect of prolactin and human placental lactogen is normally inhibited by progesterone. Fall in progesterone levels after delivery removes this inhibitory effect and promotes milk secretion.

66a. True
66b. False
66c. False – it inhibits FSH release.
66d. False – its level peaks during early pregnancy.
66e. True

67a. False
67b. False
67c. True
67d. True
67e. True

Note
Human placental lactogen (hPL) is a polypeptide hormone (consisting of 190 amino acids). Its structure and function are similar to growth hormone. It is secreted by the syncytiotrophoblast during pregnancy. The biological half-life is 15 minutes. It increases the maternal blood glucose levels and decreases its utilization (by decreasing the insulin sensitivity). Thus it promotes adequate fetal nutrition. Long-standing hypoglycaemia leads to an increase in hPL. It also promotes lipolysis and releases free fatty acids. In such situations free fatty acid is available for maternal tissues and glucose can be utilized by fetal tissues.

68a. True
68b. True
68c. True

68d. False – estriol is synthesized in the placenta from fetal precursor dehydroepiandrosterone, which in turn is converted to 16-hydroxy-dehydroepiandrosterone in the fetal liver after being secreted from the fetal adrenal gland. Estriol is formed after aromatization of the A-ring of 16-hydroxy-dehydroepiandrosterone in the placenta. Estradiol and estrone are derived from maternal precursors and also secreted from the placenta.
68e. False – testosterone is not produced in the deciduas.

69a. True
69b. True
69c. False
69d. True
69e. True

Note
The corpus luteum produces the above-mentioned hormones plus oestrogen.

70a. False – it decreases the levels of antithrombin III.
70b. False – it decreases the levels.
70c. True
70d. True
70e. False

71a. True
71b. True
71c. True
71d. False
71e. False

Note
The combined oral contraceptive pill increases the risk of pulmonary embolism, myocardial infarction and thrombotic strokes. It shows no association with trophoblastic disease and prolactinomas.

72a. True
72b. False – it inhibits oestrogen-mediated positive feedback which leads to an LH surge.
72c. False – It decreases the receptivity to the blastocyst.
72d. True
72e. False

73a. True
73b. False – post-abortion, combined pills are started the same or next day.
73c. False – day 21 in non-lactating women.
73d. False
73e. False

74a. True
74b. False – COCPs have no effect on glaucoma.
74c. False – the use of COCPs can cause cholestatic jaundice in some women.
74d. True
74e. False

75a. True
75b. True
75c. True
75d. True
75e. False

Note

There is an increase in vascularity and the size of the thyroid gland. Thyroid-binding globulin also increases.

Due to increase in GFR, the loss of iodine in the urine is increased. This loss is not reflected in the serum iodine levels unless the pregnant woman is iodine deficient (there is no reduction in the serum iodine).

76a. False – oestrogen stimulates calcitonin secretion.
76b. False – it stimulates calcitonin secretion.
76c. False – both parathyroid hormone and calcitonin regulate the calcium levels in the blood. Parathyroid hormone is a polypeptide hormone secreted by the parathyroid gland. Low calcium level in the blood (inhibits the secretion of calcitonin) stimulates the production of parathyroid hormone from the gland, which in turn mobilizes the calcium from the bone (by direct action on osteocytes) into the bloodstream. It also to some extent promotes absorption of the calcium from the gut and the kidney tubules. Calcitonin has opposite actions to parathyroid hormone and thus decreases the calcium level so that it does not rise above a certain point.
76d. True
76e. True

77a. False
77b. True
77c. True
77d. True
77e. True

Note

Anion gap is also increased in poisoning with ethylene glycol, paraldehyde and methanol whereas it is decreased with bromide poisoning.

78a. True
78b. False – it causes a decrease in the anion gap.
78c. True
78d. False
78e. True

79a. False – its concentration is proportional to PCO_2.
79b. False – it dissociates into $H_2O + CO_2$.
79c. False – it is formed from $H_2O + CO_2$.
79d. True
79e. False – H^+ ions are derived from H_2O.

80a. False
80b. True
80c. True
80d. True
80e. True

Note
It is the total number of buffer anions. A buffer solution is one where hydrogen or hydroxyl ions can be added with little change in the pH.

81a. False – there is a low PCO_2 and a high pH.
81b. True
81c. False
81d. True
81e. True

Note
It can be seen in patients with pulmonary embolus. During pregnancy there is hyperstimulation due to progesterone acting on the respiratory centre but there is no change in the pH. This is mainly due to the kidneys excreting bicarbonate and compensating for the loss of CO_2.

82a. False – alveolar air is fully saturated with water.
82b. False – alveolar ventilation is about 350 mL for each breath.
82c. True
82d. True
82e. True

83a. True
83b. False – increase in ventilation is much greater than increase in O_2 consumption.
83c. False – progesterone stimulates the respiratory centre and also increases its sensitivity to CO_2.
83d. False – the increase in ventilation is achieved by an increase in tidal volume.
83e. False

84a. True
84b. False – liquids empty before solids.
84c. False – fats are the slowest of all the emptying substances.
84d. False – isotonic contents empty before hypotonic contents.
84e. True

85a. True
85b. False
85c. True
85d. False – aortic body chemoreceptors are sensitive to changes in PCO_2 and pH.
85e. True

Note
The respiratory centre is responsible for controlling the depth as well as rhythmicity of respiration. The respiratory centre receives input from the upper medulla and also from the peripheral chemoreceptors' carotid and aortic bodies. The chemoreceptors can be stimulated by drugs such as doxapram, cyanide and nicotine. Progesterone stimulates the respiratory centre and thus causes an increase in respiratory rate.

86a. True
86b. True
86c. False – it is 10% less in women than men.
86d. False – radioactive substances are not used during pregnancy.
86e. True

Note
GFR is the clearance of a substance that is neither reabsorbed nor secreted in the renal tubule. The normal GFR is 120 mL/min. It can be measured by insulin clearance and radioactive vitamin B_{12}.

87a. False
87b. True
87c. True
87d. True
87e. True

Note
IgD helps in antigen recognition by cells.

IgM also promotes complement fixation.

88a. True
88b. True
88c. True
88d. False – there is fall in protein S levels.
88e. True

Note
There is a rise in circulating factors, e.g. fibrinogen, factors VII, VIII, IX, X, XII. Factor XI and antithrombin III levels decrease. These changes make pregnancy a hypercoagulable state.

89a. True
89b. True
89c. True

89d. False
89e. False – saturation of <15% indicates iron deficiency anaemia during pregnancy.

Note
– 70% of the total body iron is in haemoglobin.
– The maximal absorption of the iron occurs in the duodenum.
– Iron is stored as ferritin in the reticuloendothelial system.
– Iron is bound to serum-binding protein – transferrin (TIBC).
– Transferrin is mainly produced in the liver.
– Serum iron is low and TIBC is high in iron deficiency anaemia.

90a. False
90b. True – is autosomal dominant.
90c. True
90d. True
90e. True

Note
It is due to excessive deposition of haemosiderin in the tissues. This syndrome is characterized by skin pigmentation, diabetes, cirrhosis of the liver and also high predisposition to develop hepatic cancer.

91a. False
91b. True
91c. False
91d. True
91e. False

Note
Haemolytic disease of the newborn or erythroblastosis fetalis is due to Rh incompatibility where the mother produces antibodies against fetal red blood cells, RBCs (mother is rhesus negative and baby is rhesus positive). It usually does not affect the first pregnancy as the initial response to antigen on RBCs would be formation of IgM (which does not cross the placenta). In subsequent pregnancies, there is formation of IgG antibodies. The IgG antibodies can cross the placenta and, as these are against fetal RBCs, it destroys fetal RBCs (haemolysis). This can cause severe anaemia *in utero* with severe anaemia and jaundice in the newborn. If the haemolysis is severe, the baby can even die *in utero*.

The fetal haemolytic process is maximal at birth, leading to severe anaemia. At birth, the fetal conjugating system is still immature and therefore high levels of unconjugated bilirubin can accumulate in the blood, resulting in jaundice. This (bilirubin) can cross the blood–brain barrier with deposition of bilirubin in the basal ganglion, causing kernicterus.

92a. True
92b. False – red cell volume increases by 40%.
92c. True

92d. False – it reaches a plateau around 32–34 weeks.
92e. True

Note
The blood flow to various organs is increased, e.g. uterus (700 mL/min), skin (500 mL/min). There is a three-fold increase in erythropoietin levels and this is associated with an increase in red cell mass (40% rise) and also an increase in fetal haemoglobin. There is a rise in venous pressure and at the same time a fall in osmotic pressure. This contributes to the oedema during pregnancy.

93a. True
93b. False – systolic blood pressure is unchanged during pregnancy.
93c. True
93d. False – blood pressure is lower in the supine than in the sitting position.
93e. True

94a. True
94b. False – it is made of two molecules of acetylcholine.
94c. True
94d. True
94e. False – paralysis lasts longer due to abnormal pseudocholinesterase (inefficient in metabolizing the suxamethonium quickly) or no pseudocholinesterase, while the paralysis is transient in normal individuals.

95a. False – oxygen saturation is 70–80% in the umbilical vein and ductus venosus.
95b. True
95c. True
95d. False – ductus arteriosus closes due to direct effect of increasing PO_2.
95e. True

96a. True
96b. True
96c. False – decreased motility in both the small and the large intestine.
96d. True
96e. True

97a. True
97b. True
97c. False – it does not pass through the placenta.
97d. False – it is not secreted in breast milk.
97e. False

Note
Its action results from the sulphate group and protamine (cationic group) neutralizes it. It potentiates the action of antithrombin III. The dose can be monitored by APTT or factor Xa activity.

98a. False – they readily cross the placenta.
98b. False
98c. True
98d. False – it causes increase in blood pressure.
98e. True – therefore cause vomiting.

Note
Potency in terms of analgesia
Dextropropoxyphene > codeine > dihydrocodeine (>= more than).

99a. True
99b. True
99c. True
99d. False
99e. True

Note
β Agonists are used in the cases of threatened preterm labour. They should be used after excluding any contraindication, e.g. abruption, chorioamnionitis in cases of preterm premature rupture of the membranes. The RCOG recommends them for two indications: (1) until two doses of betamethasone (<36 weeks) are given; (2) intrauterine transfer to another hospital in case the neonatal facilities are not available at that gestational age in own hospital.

β Agonists increase the heart rate, cause vasodilatation and abolish the uterine contractions. The various other drugs that have been used for tocolysis include terbutaline, nifedipine, nitroglycerin patch, magnesium sulphate, indometacin and atosiban.

100a. True
100b. False – entonox is a combination of 50% oxygen and 50% nitrous oxide. It is used in labour analgesia and is not a tocolytic agent.
100c. True
100d. True
100e. True

Note
The other tocolytic agents include ritodrine and terbutaline.

101a. True
101b. True
101c. False – actinomycin D – interferes with RNA replication.
101d. False – cyclophosphamide – during interphase, it causes structural damage to the chromosomes.
101e. True

Note
Anticancer drugs are divided into various types.
1. Alkalylating agents, e.g. cyclophosphamide, melphalan and busulphan.
2. Antibiotics, e.g. doxorubicin, daunorubicin.
3. Vinca alkaloids, e.g. vincristine and vinblastine.
4. Antimetabolites, e.g. methotrexate (acts by inhibiting folic acid reductase).

5. Platinum agents, e.g. cisplatin and carboplatin. Cisplatin is both nephrotoxic and ototoxic. Carboplatin is less nephrotoxic. Both are used in the treatment of ovarian cancers.
6. Taxanes, e.g. paclitaxol (used in ovarian cancer).

102a. True
102b. True
102c. False – it causes pulmonary fibrosis.
102d. True
102e. True – both adriamycin and doxorubicin are the same drug in proprietary and generic forms.

103a. True
103b. False
103c. False
103d. True
103e. True

Note

Warfarin is teratogenic to the fetus. It is an anticoagulant and should be stopped during pregnancy due to its effects on the fetus. It can be replaced with clexane during pregnancy for maternal indications. It can cause CNS abnormalities (due to recurrent bleeds), nasal hypoplasia, chondrodysplasia punctata (stippled bone epiphysis), intrauterine growth retardation, neurodevelopmental delay, learning disability and malformations of the vertebral body (collectively called warfarin embryopathy).

104a. False – etomidate is used intravenously and is not an inhalational anaesthetic agent.
104b. True
104c. False – ketamine is used intravenously and is not an inhalational anaesthetic agent.
104d. True
104e. False – bupivacaine is a local anaesthetic agent and is commonly used for epidural analgesia.

105a. False – it is a centrally acting α_2-receptor agonist while peripherally it inhibits dopa carboxylase (methyldopa acts both centrally and peripherally).
105b. True
105c. True
105d. False – it is an antihypertensive agent and not teratogenic to the fetus. It is safe to use during pregnancy and is used as an antihypertensive agent in pre-eclampsia.
105e. True

106a. False
106b. True
106c. False
106d. True
106e. True

Note
These drugs are used in the treatment of depression and anxiety disorders. They irreversibly inhibit monoamine oxidase (MAO) enzyme in the CNS, gut and platelets. In the gut it can lead to increased absorption of tyramine, resulting in a rise in blood pressure. Patients on MAO enzyme inhibitors are normally advised to have a diet with low tyramine. It is usually advised to stop these drugs 2 weeks before surgery to prevent a hypertensive crisis due to anaesthetics. Overdose could be fatal and death may occur due to arrhythmia, renal failure or seizures. They are avoided during pregnancy because of teratogenicity.

107a. False
107b. True
107c. True
107d. False
107e. True

Note
Antipsychotic drugs are equally excreted via enterohepatic circulation in the liver as well as the kidneys. Clozepine causes agranulocytosis, so monitoring of WBCs is needed and, with low counts, it is advised to stop the medication.

Antipsychotic drugs are mainly used in the treatment of schizophrenia, bipolar disorder, psychotic symptoms, mood disorders and schizoaffective disorders.

108a. True
108b. False
108c. True
108d. True
108e. False

Note
Pro-drugs are inactive precursors that are metabolized to active metabolites in the body, e.g. cyclophosphamide becomes active after metabolism in the liver.

109a. True
109b. True
109c. True
109d. False – verapamil is extensively metabolized in the liver and about 70% of the administered dose is excreted as metabolites in urine.
109e. False – methotrexate is metabolized by intestinal bacteria to the inactive metabolite 4-amino-4-deoxy-*N*-methylpteroic acid and accounts for less than 5% loss of the oral dose. It undergoes hepatic and intracellular metabolism to the active form after its absorption. The primary route of excretion is renal (with intravenous administration about 80–90% is excreted unchanged in the urine and 10% accounts for biliary excretion). In cases of deranged renal function, its concentration in blood increases and prolongs its half-life.

110a. True
110b. True
110c. False
110d. True
110e. True

Note
Atropine, hyoscine, tropicamide and pirenzepine are muscarinic antagonists. Carbachol, bethanechol, pilocarpine and methacholine are muscarinic agonists. Both agonists and antagonists can act on the same receptor but the actions will be different. Agonists release acetylcholine and antagonists destroy acetylcholine.

111a. True
111b. False
111c. True
111d. False
111e. True

Note
Pilocarpine, timolol, clonidine, acetazolamide and dorzolamide lower the intraocular pressure. Acetazolamide is a carbonic anhydrase inhibitor and timolol is a β-adrenoreceptor antagonist.

112a. False – lactulose is an osmotic agent.
112b. True
112c. False – liquid paraffin is a faecal softener.
112d. True
112e. False – is a stimulant.

113a. False – it is a polypeptide that is prepared from bovine lung.
113b. True
113c. False – it inhibits plasmin and plasminogen activators.
113d. False
113e. True

Note
ε-Aminocaproic acid, tranexamic acid (used in the treatment of menorrhagia) and aprotinin are antifibrinolytic agents. They can cause thrombosis (aprotinin less than ε-aminocaproic acid).

114a. False – irreversibly and covalently bind to the enzyme cyclooxygenase.
114b. False – it causes reduction in the thromboxane A_2 production in platelets.
114c. False – undergoes first-pass metabolism in the liver (around 50%).
114d. False – higher doses (analgesic dose) have this effect.
114e. True

115a. False – it can cause tachycardia.
115b. True
115c. False – it causes water intoxication due to its antidiuretic effect.
115d. True
115e. False

116a. True
116b. False
116c. True
116d. False – it can cause an increase in blood pressure.
116e. True

117a. False
117b. True
117c. True
117d. True
117e. False – perinatal death rate is the number of stillbirths plus first week deaths per 1000 live births and stillbirths.

118a. False
118b. False
118c. True
118d. True
118e. True

Note
Early neonatal deaths are deaths that occur between 0 and 6 days of life. Early neonatal death rate is the number of deaths at 0–6 days per 1000 live births. Late neonatal deaths are deaths occurring between 7 and 27 days of life. Late neonatal death rate is the number of deaths at 7–27 days per 1000 live births. Neonatal deaths are deaths occurring between 0 and 27 days of life. Neonatal death rate is the number of deaths occurring between 0 and 27 days per 1000 live births.

Postneonatal deaths are deaths after 28 days of life and less than (<) 1 year of life.

Postneonatal death rate is the number of deaths >28 days but <1 year per 1000 live births.

119a. True
119b. True
119c. False – the risk of pneumonia is 10% with primary varicella-zoster (VZ) infection during pregnancy.
119d. False – the risk of congenital varicella syndrome is 2% with maternal VZ infection <20 weeks.
119e. True

120a. True
120b. True
120c. False – prevalence = incidence × time.
120d. True
120e. True

121a. True
121b. True
121c. True
121d. True
121e. True

Note
Data can be described numerically or graphically by summarizing what is observed in the sample, e.g. population. This is called descriptive statistics and the descriptors include mean and standard deviation for continuous data, e.g. weight and height, whilst the term categorical data is used to describe parameters such as race in a population (frequency and percentage).

122a. False
122b. False
122c. True
122d. True
122e. True

Note
Sensitivity is the ability of a test to correctly identify patients who have a disease.
Specificity is the ability of a test to correctly identify patients who do not have disease.

Positive predictive value (PPV) is the proportion of patients with positive test results who are correctly diagnosed.

Negative predictive value (NPV) is the proportion of patients with negative test result who are correctly diagnosed.

PPV and NPV depend on the prevalence of the disease.

123a. True
123b. True
123c. True
123d. True
123e. True

Note
Screening test: tests (e.g. cervical smear, blood tests, clinical examinations and procedures) that are used to screen healthy people to identify an unrecognized disease or condition. It is not a diagnostic test. The people who are screen positive will need further investigations in order to make a diagnosis and undertake treatment if needed.

124a. True
124b. False – it is the ratio of the risk in an exposed group to that in the unexposed group.
124c. False – RR = 1 means that there is no exposure–outcome association.
124d. True
124e. False

Note
RR < 1 means that there is decreased risk or association between exposure and outcome.

125a. False
125b. False
125c. True
125d. False
125e. True

Note
Relative risk (RR): the ratio of probability of outcome in one group of people compared with another group.
RR < 1 means decreased risk between exposure and outcome.
RR = 1 means no difference in risk between exposure and outcome.
RR > 1 means increased risk between exposure and outcome.
Risk ratio: the ratio of risk of events/outcome or side effects occurring in exposed or experimental group compared with control group.

126a. False – a retrospective longitudinal study.
126b. True
126c. True
126d. False – it requires a small number of patients and controls.
126e. True

127a. False – randomized controlled studies are a type of parallel study.
127b. True
127c. True
127d. True
127e. True

Note
Parallel studies: these are prospective longitudinal studies (these observe a process over a period of time to investigate changes) performed during the later phases of the evaluation of interventions, where the intervention under investigation is directly compared with the standard treatment or placebo.

Randomized controlled trials are the gold standard of clinical research. These are parallel studies, where patients are randomly allocated to intervention and standard treatment or placebo. There can be two or more than two arms in the study.

Randomization is a method based on chance by which study participants are assigned to a treatment group.

128a. False – it is defined as blood loss of >500 mL after vaginal delivery.
128b. True
128c. True
128d. False – trauma is seen in 7% of the cases of PPH.
128e. True

129a. True
129b. False
129c. False
129d. False
129e. False

Note
Low birth weight (LBW), weight <2500 g. Very low birth weight (VLBW), weight <1500 g. Extremely low birth weight (ELBW), weight <1000 g.

130a. True
130b. False – it gives rise to the anterior belly of digastric.
130c. True
130d. False – second arch or hyoid arch gives rise to stapedius.
130e. False – third arch gives rise to stylopharyngeus.

Note
The first pharyngeal arch is also called the mandibular arch. It gives rise to muscles that include temporalis, masseter, medial and lateral pterygoids, anterior belly of digastric, tensor palati and tensor tympani. The maxillary and mandibular divisions of the trigeminal nerve supply the muscles arising from the first arch.

It also gives rise to skeletal structures including the sphenomandibular ligament, ligament of malleus, Meckel cartilage, part of the temporal bone, zygomatic bone, mandible, maxilla, malleus and incus.

131a. False
131b. True
131c. False
131d. True
131e. True

Note
Type I pneumocytes are squamous cells lining the alveoli and help in gaseous exchange.

Surfactant is synthesized by type 2 pneumocytes in the alveoli. It reduces the surface tension and helps in expansion of the lungs. The inability of the immature lungs to synthesize surfactant in adequate amounts in preterm babies can result in respiratory distress syndrome (RDS).

132a. True
132b. False – labia minora are lined by stratified squamous epithelium (keratinized) on the lateral surface and mucous membrane on the inside.
132c. True

132d. True
132e. True

Note
The ectocervix is lined by non-keratinized, stratified, squamous epithelium while the endocervix is lined by columnar or glandular epithelium.

133a. True
133b. False
133c. True
133d. True
133e. True

Note
Bacteria are small organisms (0.3–2.0 μm). They are prokaryotic cells and contain a nucleoid region but no nuclear membrane. They contain both DNA and RNA and replicate by binary fission (asexual). They contain ribosomes but do not contain any membrane-bound organelles.

On the other hand, viruses are minute organisms (0.02–0.30 μm), except poxvirus. They do not have a cell wall, ribosomes or mitochondria. They are obligate intracellular pathogens (i.e. can replicate only in living cells) and use host organelles. They consist of a core of nucleic acid, either DNA or RNA, with a protein shell called a capsid.

134a. False – is not an obligate intracellular pathogen.
134b. False – is not an obligate intracellular pathogen.
134c. True
134d. True
134e. True

135a. False – is a lipopolysaccharide.
135b. False – is heat stable.
135c. True
135d. False – it cannot be modified by heat or chemicals.
135e. False

Note
Endotoxin (lipopolysaccharide) is part of the outer membrane of Gram-negative organisms. It is heat stable (cannot be modified by either heat or chemicals). It is not strongly immunogenic and therefore not convertible to a toxoid, unlike exotoxins (can be modified by heat or chemicals to form toxoid and can be used as a vaccine). Endotoxins activate macrophages and promote release of TNF-α and interleukin-1 and interleukin-6. This leads to tissue damage.

Exotoxins are protein substances and secreted by certain bacterial Gram-negative and Gram-positive organisms. These substances are responsible for lysis of cells by damaging cell membranes.

136a. True
136b. True
136c. True
136d. True
136e. True

Note
Exotoxins can have a different mechanism of action and therefore act at various sites in the body, e.g. *Clostridium tetani* produces neurotoxin and inhibits the release of the inhibitory neurotransmitters glycine and GABA, and therefore inhibits transmission in inhibitory synapses. On the other hand, *Clostridium botulinum* inhibits the release of acetylcholine and therefore inhibits cholinergic synapses. *Clostridium perfringens* produces an α-toxin (lecithinase) and causes cytolysis (causes cell membrane damage leading to myonecrosis).

Exotoxin A produced by *Pseudomonas aeruginosa* causes ADP ribosylation and inactivation of elongation factor 2, resulting in inhibition of protein synthesis and cell death. Diphtheria toxin produced by *Corynebacterium diphtheriae* acts in a similar way to exotoxin A. These also cause lysis of cells.

137a. False – it is an endotoxin released by the outer membrane of Gram-negative organisms.
137b. True
137c. True
137d. False – it is a neurotoxin that inhibits release of the inhibitory neurotransmitters glycine and GABA.
137e. False

Note
The exotoxins that cause inhibition of protein synthesis in eukaryotic cells are diphtheria toxin (produced by *Corynebacterium diphtheriae*), exotoxin A (produced by *Pseudomonas aeruginosa*), shigella toxin (produced by *Shigella dysenteriae*) and verotoxin (produced by enterohaemorrhagic *E. coli*).

Vibrio cholerae produces a heat-labile toxin. It causes stimulation of adenylyl cyclase by ADP ribosylation of GTP-binding protein. This promotes loss of electrolytes and fluids from the intestine, leading to profuse watery diarrhoea.

138a. False – is an obligate aerobic bacterium.
138b. False – is an obligate aerobic bacterium.
138c. False – is a microaerophilic organism.
138d. True
138e. True

Note
Obligate aerobes – need O_2.

Obligate anaerobes – cannot use O_2.

Facultative anaerobes – use O_2 until finished and then either ferment or respire anaerobically.

Microaerophilic – requires low oxygen tension.

139a. False
139b. True
139c. False
139d. True
139e. True

Note

S. aureus produces various enzymes (coagulase, staphylokinase and hyaluronidase) and exotoxins. It is a Gram-positive coccus and seen in clusters. It is part of the normal flora of the skin and nasal mucosa. It can spread via hands and sneezing. The various staphylococcal species include: *S. aureus*, *S. epidermidis* (coagulase negative) and *S. saprophyticus*. *S. aureus* can cause abscesses (boils and carbuncles), food poisoning, toxic shock syndrome, pneumonia, impetigo and gastroenteritis. *S. epidermidis* can cause intravenous catheter-related infections.

Meticillin-resistant *S. aureus* (MRSA), as the name suggests, is generally resistant to almost all antibiotics except vancomycin and fusidic acid. Topical mupirocin is used in patients or staff who carry this organism in their nasal mucosa. In the UK, one needs to follow respective hospital policy for MRSA.

Streptococcus is also a Gram-positive coccus and is seen in pairs or chains. They are catalase negative. They are classified according to their appearance on blood agar as α-haemolytic, β-haemolytic (further classified into Lancefield groups as group A and group B) and non-haemolytic.

For example, the β-haemolytic group A streptococcus, *S. pyogenes*, causes spreading cellulitis, tonsillitis, pharyngitis and scarlet fever. It can cause rheumatic fever and acute glomerulonephritis. It is also a recognized cause of puerperal sepsis and neonatal septicaemia. Pregnant women who carry group B streptococci in the vagina receive prophylactic benzylpenicillin (3 g stat intravenous dose and 1.2 g four hourly until the delivery of the baby) in labour to prevent transmission of this organism to the fetus.

S. agalactiae is a β-haemolytic, group B streptococcus.

S. viridans is an α-haemolytic streptococcus – causes bacterial endocarditis.

140a. True
140b. True
140c. True
140d. False – Its capsule contains a polypeptide.
140e. True

Note

B. anthracis is a Gram-positive spore-forming rod and produces exotoxin. Animals, skin and soil are the reservoirs of this organism. The spores survive long after the animal dies. It causes cutaneous anthrax (papules with vesicles are seen on the skin associated with painful regional lymphadenopathy) and wool-sorter's disease (life-threatening pneumonia). Anthrax disease is common in animals and rare in humans. It can be transmitted to humans if someone comes in contact with affected animals or inhales the spores.

141a. True
141b. True
141c. False
141d. False
141e. False

Note
The following arise from ectoderm:
Epidermis
Hair, nail and enamel of teeth
Mammary gland
Cerebral hypophysis
Sensory epithelia of the nose, eyes and ears
Brain and spinal cord
Also structures arising from neuroectoderm (neural crest cells).

The following arise from endoderm:
Epithelial lining of the tympanic cavity, tympanic antrum and auditory tube
Epithelial lining of urinary bladder
Epithelial lining of respiratory tract
Epithelial lining of gastrointestinal tract
Thymus, thyroid and parathyroid gland.

The following arise from mesoderm:
Smooth and striated muscle
Cartilage and bones
Spleen, kidneys and heart
Blood and lymph vessels
Ovaries, testes and genital ducts (somatic tissues of the ovaries)
Cortex of suprarenal gland.

142a. False
142b. True
142c. False
142d. True
142e. True

Note
In addition to the functions mentioned in Question 142, skin acts as a protective barrier against shearing forces and helps to feel touch, pain and temperature. It promotes wound healing and synthesizes vitamin D (ultraviolet induced).

143a. True
143b. False
143c. False – it is usually associated with orofacial lesions and encephalitis. It also affects the genital area.
143d. True
143e. True

Note
HSV is a DNA virus. HSVs are of two types (type 1 and type 2). Type 1 HSV usually causes cold sores (which can be recurrent as the virus remains latent in

dorsal root ganglia and trigeminal ganglia) and ocular lesions, and can also cause genital lesions in 50% of cases (orogenital contact). The cell-mediated immunity develops after the infection. It can cause recurrent attacks in individuals with immunosuppression and HIV. It can autoinnoculate into areas of trauma and present as painful blisters (herpetic whitlow).

Type 2 usually causes genital lesions. It is sexually transmitted and often, symptomatic and causes painful vesicles in the genital area (primary genital herpes), with fever, myalgia and autonomic neuropathy (causing bladder atony and retention of urine). This may need catheterization and hospitalization. The incubation period is 3 weeks. Anti-HSV antibodies form after an attack and recurrent attacks could be less severe, of shorter duration with fewer constitutional symptoms and less viral shedding in the presence of anti-HSV antibodies. Asymptomatic shedding of the virus can also occur.

It can cause other complications including corneal ulceration, erythema multiforme and eczema herpeticum.

During pregnancy, HSV may cause fetal infection in the perinatal period. Most infection in neonates occurs if the infection in the mother is a primary, i.e. first time, genital HSV infection and is transmitted to the fetus during its travel through the birth canal. The risk of transmission to the fetus or neonate is much lower (around 3%) with recurrent herpes due to transfer of passive immunity.

Caesarean section is recommended in women if the primary attack of genital HSV infection is within 6 weeks of labour or lesions are visible at the time of labour (there is no benefit of caesarean section if the membranes have ruptured for more than 4 hours). Paediatricians need to be informed as it can cause serious infections in the neonate including disseminated disease (mortality rate = 70–80%). It can cause life-threatening pneumonia and encephalitis (mortality rate >90%) in the newborn with long-term sequelae.

The Tzank test is used to demonstrate multinucleate giant cells. Also swabs from vesicle fluid can be taken for culture. Treatment of genital lesions is mainly supportive (pain relief and treatment of secondary infection). Oral aciclovir (200 mg five times a day for 5 days) is used in cases of primary genital HSV and this may shorten the duration of symptoms.

144a. True
144b. False
144c. False
144d. True
144e. False

Note
It is a common skin infection of childhood. It presents as multiple, small, umbilicated (the lesions have a central depression called a punctum), solid lesions on skin (<0.5 cm) and can occur anywhere in the body. Occasionally, they can reach 1 cm in size and are called giant molluscum. The spread is by direct contact and scratching promotes its spread. As they resolve spontaneously, they rarely require treatment.

A skin lesion appearing along the lines of trauma is called the Koebner phenomenon.

145a. True
145b. True
145c. True
145d. False – the incidence of Down syndrome is 1:100 at the age of 40 years.
145e. False – the incidence of Down syndrome is 1:40 at the age of 44 years and 1:31 at the age of 45 years.

Note
The screening tests that are used for Down syndrome in the second trimester (from 15 weeks onwards) include:

Double test – utilizes serum βhCG (human chorionic gonadotrophin) and AFP (α-fetoprotein).
Triple test – utilizes serum βhCG, AFP and uE_3 (estriol).
Quadruple test – utilizes serum βhCG, AFP, uE_3 and inhibin.

Down syndrome is associated with high βhCG, low AFP and low uE_3.

The screening tests that are used for Down syndrome in the first trimester include:

Nuchal translucency: the fluid at the back of the neck measured under ultrasound guidance (performed between 11 and 14 weeks).
Serum markers – PAPP-A (pregnancy-associated plasma protein A) and βhCG.

146a. True
146b. True
146c. True
146d. True
146e. True

Note
Odds – the probability of the event occurring compared with that of not occurring.
Odds = probability/(1 – probability).
Odds ratio – the ratio of odds of events occurring in an experimental group when compared with the control group.
Odds ratio < 1 means decreased risk between exposure and outcome.
Odds ratio $= 1$ means no difference in risk between exposure and outcome.
Odds ratio > 1 means increased risk between exposure and outcome.

147a. True
147b. False
147c. False
147d. True
147e. True

Note
Direct – deaths resulting from obstetric complications of the pregnant state (pregnancy, labour and puerperium), from interventions, omissions, incorrect treatment, or from a chain of events resulting from any of the above.

Indirect – deaths resulting from previous existing disease, or disease that developed during pregnancy and that was not due to direct obstetric causes, but was aggravated by the physiological effects of pregnancy.

Late – deaths occurring between 42 days and 1 year after abortion, miscarriage or delivery that are due to direct or indirect maternal causes.

Coincidental or fortuitous – deaths from unrelated causes that happen to occur in pregnancy or the puerperium

Reference:
Lewis, G (ed). The Confidential Enquiry into Maternal and Child Health (CEMACH). *Saving Mothers' Lives: reviewing maternal deaths to make motherhood safer – 2003–2005. The Seventh Report on Confidential Enquiries into Maternal Deaths in the United Kingdom*. London: CEMACH, 2007. Available at: www.cmace.org.uk.

148a. True – statistical summation of results from studies conducted on specific clinical condition. The results are usually presented with *p* values and confidence intervals (CIs).
148b. True
148c. True
148d. False – patients in one trial are not directly compared with those in another trial. Each trial is analysed separately. Summary statistics are added together in the meta-analysis.
148e. True

Note
Systematic review is a scientific evaluation of several studies conducted on a specific clinical condition. They are mostly conducted on randomized controlled trials but also on other studies.

149a. True
149b. False
149c. True
149d. False
149e. True

Note
Placebo effect: results from the belief that one is being treated rather than having actual treatment effect (physiological, physical or chemical actions or activities of the treatment).

Double blind: neither the subjects being treated nor the people evaluating the outcome variables know which treatment the subjects are receiving.

150a. True
150b. False
150c. False
150d. True
150e. False

Note
Null hypothesis
– States that no relationship exists between the variables and outcome of the study.
– Any observed association occurs by chance (presumed answer to any scientific question until proved otherwise).

The *p* value
– Is used to accept or reject the null hypothesis in a study.
– Significant results are those unlikely to have occurred by chance, thus rejecting the null hypothesis.
– Non-significant results are those where a chance occurrence has not been ruled out, thus the null hypothesis has not been disproved.
– $p < 0.05$ (probability of obtaining a result by chance is <1:20) is the accepted threshold for a statistical significance or minimum evidence needed to discard the null hypothesis.

Type II error
– Occurs when the null hypothesis is not rejected when it is false.
– For example, failing to find a significant result ($p > 0.05$) between the samples when it really exists.

Type I error
– Occurs when the null hypothesis is rejected when it is actually true.
– For example, there is significant difference ($p < 0.05$) between the samples when it is actually not true.
– An alternative hypothesis specifies a real value for a parameter that will be considered when the null hypothesis is rejected.

151a. True
151b. True
151c. True
151d. False
151e. True

Note
Transplacental – cytomegalovirus, *Toxoplasma*, syphilis, *Listeria*, rubella, parvovirus and HIV.
Breast milk – HIV, *S. aureus*.
Birth canal – group B streptococci, *Chlamydia*, gonorrhoea, herpes simplex virus, human papillomavirus.

152a. False – more common in newborn babies born before 34 weeks.
152b. False – less common in newborn babies born after 36 weeks.
152c. True
152d. True
152e. True

153a. False
153b. False
153c. False
153d. False
153e. False

Notes
Hepatitis E virus is a single-stranded RNA virus and belongs to the calcivirus family. It is enterically transmitted and is not blood borne. It does not cause chronic liver disease. Pregnant women with hepatitis E infection can develop fulminant hepatic failure (mortality rate 5%).

154a. False
154b. True – it is a single-stranded RNA virus.
154c. True
154d. True
154e. False – Koplik spots are pathognomic for measles or rubeola (caused by paramyxoviruses).

Note
German measles or rubella is an acute and highly infectious disease. It is an RNA togavirus and is transmitted by respiratory droplet infection. The individual presents with constitutional symptoms (fever, arthralgia) and maculopapular rash with suboccipital and postauricular lymphadenopathy. The incubation period is 2–3 weeks and the affected individual is infectious 1 week after the appearance of the rash and also during the last week of the incubation period. The first response is formation of IgM antibodies which usually disappear within 2–3 months.

It is transmitted to the fetus, transplacentally. The risk of transmission to the fetus with associated congenital anomalies is highest if the mother acquires infection during the first trimester and decreases thereafter (>80% in the first 4 weeks, 25% in the next 4 weeks and 10% from 8 to 12 weeks). The risk is less than 10% with re-infection.

The associated defects in the fetus are attributed to vascular damage or reduced mitotic activity. It can cause cardiac defect, sensorineural deafness, cataract, microcephaly and learning disability. Splenomegaly, purpura, jaundice, meningoencephalitis and thrombocytopenia could be transient features seen in the newborn. The late-onset features are diabetes, precocious puberty and progressive panencephalitis.

Attenuated MMR (measles mumps rubella) vaccine is give at 18 months of age for the prevention of the disease. It is contraindicated during pregnancy as there is a small risk of congenital rubella syndrome. Women who are not immune and have been tested for rubella IgG antibody during pregnancy should be vaccinated postpartum and advised to avoid contact with other women and children with German measles.

155a. True
155b. False
155c. True

155d. False
155e. True

Note
Rickettsia rickettsii contains both DNA and RNA and divides by binary fission. It contains a Gram-negative cell envelope. It cannot create its own energy (ATP) and therefore is unable to grow in cell-free medium. Wild rodents are the reservoir of this bacterium and it is transmitted by the bite of hard ticks. It invades the endothelial lining of the capillaries and causes vasculitis. It causes the disease Rocky Mountain spotted fever (presents with headache, raised temperature, myalgia, vomiting, confusion and maculopapular rash). The incubation period is a few days to 2 weeks. The diagnosis can be made by the Weil–Felix test or complement fixation test. The organism is sensitive to tetracycline (e.g. doxycycline) and erythromycin.

156a. False
156b. True
156c. True
156d. True
156e. False

Note
Infectious mononucleosis is caused by Epstein–Barr virus (belongs to herpes virus). It is rare in young children and more common between 14 and 18 years of age. The clinical presentation is severe malaise, pharyngitis, fever and lymphadenopathy. Treatment is usually symptomatic. A rash develops on administration of ampicillin.

157a. False
157b. True
157c. True
157d. False
157e. False

Note
Human papillomavirus (HPV) is a double-stranded DNA virus. It can be transmitted sexually and has a predilection to affect squamous epithelium, resulting in cellular transformation. This involves loss of maturation in the squamous epithelium (transformation to less differentiated cell type) of the cervix.

Its viral genome is made of early (E) and late (L) regions. The early region contains eight open reading frames (ORFs), which code proteins responsible for viral maintenance and replication. The late region has two ORFs, which produce proteins that form the viral capsid. Integration of the virus into the host cell DNA plays an important role in the development of cervical intra-epithelial neoplasia (CIN) and cervical cancer.

HPV is present in $>$99% of cervical cancer. There is considerable evidence that HPV is necessary for the development of the majority of cervical cancer and its precursor lesion, CIN. HPV infection can be sexually transmitted; women carrying this virus are usually asymptomatic and the infection may be transient. However, if the HPV virus persists in the cervix, then it may lead to high-grade CIN and ultimately cervical cancer. In the UK, HPV type 16 accounts for 60–80% of high-grade CIN and cervical cancer. The remainder are mostly caused by HPV types 18, 31, 33 and 35. HPV6 and -11 (low risk types) cause benign viral warts. The high-risk HPVs are types 16, 18, 31, 33, 35, 39, 45, 51, 52, 56 and 58.

Prevention of cervical cancer is the best strategy if possible. This could be achieved in two ways: (1) taking measures to avoid the risk factors (early age of intercourse, multiple sexual partners, smoking, etc.) leading to development of CIN and cervical cancer. (2) Early detection of precancerous abnormalities of the cervix (CIN) and treatment. One way to achieve the second option is to remove the whole transformation zone (excisional form of treatment of CIN) to treat CIN and eradicate HPV. The success rate of this treatment is 95%. The latest innovation is the HPV vaccine to prevent CIN and cervical cancer.

158a. True
158b. False
158c. True
158d. False
158e. True

Note
Viruses can contain either DNA or RNA. The DNA-containing viruses are herpes viruses (herpes virus type 1, herpes virus type 2, varicella-zoster virus, cytomegalovirus and Epstein–Barr virus), adenoviruses, poxviruses (smallpox, vaccinia, molluscum contagiosum), hepatitis B virus and papovaviruses.

The viruses that contain RNA are retroviruses (HIV-1, HIV-2 and HTLV-1), rhabdoviruses (rabies), picornaviruses (enteroviruses – polio virus, hepatitis A virus, echovirus and rhinovirus – common cold virus), reoviruses, myxoviruses (influenza A, B, C), paramyxoviruses (parainfluenza, mumps, measles, respiratory syncytial virus), arboviruses (dengue, yellow fever and sandfly fever) and togavirus (rubella – single-stranded small RNA virus).

159a. True – Spiral bacterium.
159b. False – Is sensitive to drying and water.
159c. False – Does not grow in culture.
159d. True – It is visualized by dark-ground microscopy or fluorescent antibody technique.
159e. False – May cross placenta after 16 weeks of pregnancy.

Note
Treponema pallidum infection spreads by direct sexual contact and spreads in the body through the bloodstream and lymphatics. It can be diagnosed by Venereal Disease Reference Laboratory (VDRL) test (tests reagin antibody and not very specific as it can be positive in various other infections) and specific tests such as *Treponema pallidum* haemagglutination assay (TPHA – detects IgG antibody and remains positive after treatment for many years), fluorescent treponemal antibody absorbed test (FTA-abs), ELISA and *Treponema pallidum* immobilization test.

160a. False
160b. True – Carbol fuchsin stain is used in this method.
160c. True – It also resists decolorization by acid and is therefore called acid and alchohol fast.
160d. False
160e. True – Contains glycerol and egg yolk.

Note
The tubercle bacillus was first discovered in 1882 by Robert Koch. It is an aerobic (requires O_2) bacterium and is resistant to drying and also to stains unless heated. It has a waxy coating on the cell surface and is made of mycolic acid (lipid). This is probably responsible for its resistance and contributes to virulence. It grows slowly in culture, taking 6 weeks (divides every 15–20 hours).

In lungs, it is taken up by alveolar macrophages but they are unable to destroy this organism. A typical lesion is a caseating granuloma (consisting of macrophages with central caseation). It is acquired by the respiratory route as a result of close contact with somebody infected with tuberculosis of the lung. The primary focus or Ghon focus usually begins in the upper lobe of the lung. It can spread to the lymph nodes or any organ in the body via the bloodstream, leading to military tuberculosis. It is associated with cell-mediated immunity, on which the Mantoux and Heaf tests (skin tests) are based.

161a. True – This enzyme helps in synthesis of DNA from its RNA. This DNA is then incorporated into the host cell genome.
161b. False – It is a retrovirus and contains RNA.
161c. True – Reverse transcriptase promotes this process.
161d. True – It recognizes the CD4 receptor molecule and then gains entry into the T-helper cells. Ultimately these cells are destroyed.
161e. True

162a. False
162b. True
162c. False – Needs 5% CO_2 to grow.
162d. True – Thayer–Martin medium is used for culture of this organism.
162e. False – Is a late complication.

Note
N. gonorrhoeae is a Gram-negative diplococcus. This organism can be seen within the cytoplasm of polymorphs on Gram staining. It can cause urethritis (males) and cervicitis (females), proctitis, pharyngitis and septic arthritis. It can also cause conjunctivitis in the newborn (acquired during its passage through the birth canal).

163a. True – It is a spirochaetal organism.
163b. False – It is transmitted by tick bite (*Ixodes dammini*).
163c. True – Rash develops at the site of the tick bite (annular rash with central clearing and a raised red border).
163d. False – It is not associated with granuloma formation.
163e. True

Note
Other symptoms are fever, headache, myalgia, arthralgia, lymphadenopathy and malaise.

164a. True – also called fifth disease.
164b. True – it is associated with arthralgia.
164c. True – causes red cell aplasia.
164d. True
164e. True – slapped-cheek appearance.

165a. True
165b. False – causes granuloma formation. It has a predilection for skin and cutaneous nerves.
165c. True
165d. False
165e. False – carbol fuchsin dye is used for staining.

Note
M. leprae (aerobic rod-shaped bacillus) is the causative organism of leprosy (Hansen disease). It is an obligate intracellular parasite and has an outer waxy coat made of mycolic acid. It is mostly found in warm tropical countries.

It is seen in clumps on optical microscopy and has been successfully grown in mouse footpads and armadillos. It replicates very slowly and is difficult to culture in artificial cell culture media. It is sensitive to dapsone, rifampicin and clofazimine. WHO recommends multi-drug treatment rather than single agent therapy as dapsone resistance has developed over time.

166a. False – it belongs to the hepadnavirus family.
166b. True – it has reverse transcriptase activity.
166c. True
166d. False – it is composed of protein (polypeptide).
166e. True – it is one of the few non-retroviruses that uses reverse transcription for its replication.

167a. True
167b. False
167c. True
167d. False
167e. False

Note
Trichomonas vaginalis (TV) is a single-celled, flagellated, motile protozoan. It is slightly larger than a granulocyte and depends on adherence to the host cell for its survival. Women can present with yellowish-green frothy vaginal discharge (has odour), itching of the genital area, dysuria and dyspareunia (vaginitis, cervicitis and urethritis). It may lead to premature rupture of membranes and preterm delivery. It can coexist with other genital infections such as gonorrhoea, *Chlamydia* and bacterial vaginosis. Most men are usually asymptomatic and can (rarely) develop genital irritation, epididymitis and prostatitis.

On speculum examination, the vaginal mucosa is erythematous and the cervix is inflamed with numerous petechiae (strawberry appearance). Motile organisms are seen on wet-mount saline preparation under the microscope. Wet-mount microscopy and culture are the gold standard for its diagnosis. Metronidazole is the drug of choice for treatment.

168a. True
168b. False
168c. True
168d. False
168e. True

Note

Bacterial vaginosis (BV) is a polymicrobial superficial vaginal infection due to an overgrowth of anaerobes and is the most common cause of vaginal discharge. *Gardnerella vaginalis* (also known as *Haemophilus vaginalis*) is a facultative, anaerobic, non-flagellated, non-spore-forming bacterium. It is recognized as one of the organisms responsible for causing bacterial vaginosis. The other organisms involved in this pathology are *Bacteroides*, *Peptostreptococcus*, *Fusobacterium*, *Mycoplasma hominis*, *Mobiluncus* and *Veilonella*.

Women present with thin grey homogeneous vaginal discharge and a characteristic fishy odour (alkalinity of semen may cause a release of volatile amines from the vaginal discharge – forms the basis for the whiff test). The fishy smell is mainly recognized after sexual intercourse. Vulval itching, dysuria and dyspareunia are rare. It is also known to cause vault infection following hysterectomy and pelvic infection after abortion. In pregnant women it has been associated with premature rupture of membranes and preterm delivery. The following are recognized as risk factors for the development of BV: vaginal douching, antibiotic use, decrease in oestrogen production, presence of intrauterine device and increase in number of sexual partners.

There is an increase in vaginal pH as it is associated with a decrease in lactobacilli (responsible for maintaining the acidic pH) in the vagina. Wet-mount saline preparation with vaginal discharge shows clue cells (vaginal epithelial cells have a stippled appearance due to adherence of coccobacilli) under low and high power microscopy. The drug used for treatment is metronidazole (single dose of 2 g or 7-day course of oral dose (500 mg bd for 7 days)). Metronidazole is contraindicated during early pregnancy. Topical clindamycin and metronidazole are also useful in returning the vaginal flora to normal.

Amsel's criteria for diagnosis of bacterial vaginosis are: (a) thin white homogeneous discharge; (b) increase in vaginal pH (>4.5); (c) clue cells on microscopy; and (d) whiff test – when a few drops of alkali (10% KOH) are added to vaginal secretions, a fishy smell is released. At least three of the four criteria should be present to make the diagnosis.

169a. False – It is an obligate intracellular pathogen and cannot grow outside a living cell.
169b. True
169c. True
169d. True
169e. True

Note
Chlamydia infection is a sexually transmitted infection. Certain strains of *Chlamydia trachomatis* (serovars A, B, Ba, C) are associated with trachoma, which is a major cause of blindness worldwide. Serovars L1, L2 and L3 are associated with lymphogranuloma venereum. Serovars D to K cause non-specific urethritis and epididymitis in men and perihepatitis, cervicitis, urethritis, endometritis and salpingitis (infection of upper genital tract – leading to PID) in women. It can cause Reiter syndrome in both men and women (conjunctivitis, proctitis, urethritis and reactive seronegative arthritis). Its long-term sequelae include chronic pelvic pain, infertility and ectopic pregnancy. It is associated with increased rates of transmission of HIV infection. It can be transmitted to the neonate during its passage through the birth canal and may cause conjunctivitis and pneumonia.

The incubation period is 1–3 weeks and men present with mucopurulent urethral discharge (urethritis) and women present with vaginal discharge (cervicitis). Asymptomatic infection is not uncommon in both men and women. Cervical or urethral swabs (first sample of urine in men) are collected for culture and nucleic acid amplification test. It is sensitive to doxycycline and erythromycin group of drugs.

170a. True
170b. False
170c. True
170d. True
170e. True

Note
Methyldopa is an antihypertensive agent and is absorbed from the gut. It is metabolized in the liver and intestine. Its metabolite, α-methylnorepinephrine, stimulates the α_2-adrenergic receptors in the brain, leading to decrease in the peripheral resistance (negative feedback effect on the sympathetic nervous system both centrally and peripherally causing its tone to reduce). It is used as a first-line antihypertensive agent in pregnant women unless there is a history of hypersensitive reaction. It needs to be stopped after delivery and changed to another antihypertensive agent if needed as it is known to cause postnatal depression.

Various side effects such as postural hypotension, sedation, dizziness, headache, myalgia, bradycardia, depression, hepatitis, abnormal liver function tests, hyperprolactinaemia and lupus-like syndrome have been reported.

171a. False
171b. True
171c. True
171d. False
171e. True

Note
Gap junction synchronizes the myometrial function via conduction of electrophysiological stimuli during labour. Oestrogen and prostaglandin induce gap junctions.

172a. True
172b. False – causes increase in the number of oxytocin receptors.
172c. True
172d. False – it induces gap junctions and increases their number.
172e. False – progesterone causes this action.

173a. False – induces uterine contractions at all gestational ages when administered externally.
173b. True
173c. False – PGE_2 and PGF_2 are produced by the placenta, chorion, amnion and decidua. They are required for the onset of labour and are found in increasing amounts before the onset.
173d. True
173e. True

Note
Prostaglandin production increases in uterine tissue during pregnancy. It is used in cervical ripening and induction of labour. The concentration also increases in amniotic fluid and maternal blood. It induces gap junction and stimulates uterine contractions during labour (natural or induced). The following stimulate synthesis of PGE_2 in fetal membranes: infection, hypoxia, prostaglandins and oxytocin administration.

174a. True
174b. True
174c. False
174d. False
174e. True

Note
β Agonists used for tocolysis for preterm labour are non-selective and therefore act on both β_1 and β_2 receptors. β_2 Agonists act on the receptors located on the myocytes and initiate myometrial relaxation by stimulation of cAMP. This reduces the calcium influx along with inhibition of the myosin light-chain kinase. Examples are ritodrine, salbutamol and terbutaline.

The side effects are tremor, palpitations, headache, tachycardia and serious complications such as pulmonary oedema. β-Receptor stimulation also leads to vasodilatation and as a result there is a compensatory tachycardia, increase in stroke volume and increase in the cardiac output.

Stimulation of β_2 receptors causes glycogenolysis and elevation in the blood sugar levels, while β_1-receptor stimulation causes mobilization of free fatty acids and glycolysis. The above actions explain the indications for contraindications.

On the other hand, the calcium channel blocker nifedipine inhibits the calcium influx across the cell membranes and therefore reduces the tone of the smooth muscle cells in the uterus.

175a. True
175b. False – increases uterine blood flow by myometrial relaxation.
175c. True
175d. True – lipid-soluble drugs such as ritodrine can cross the placenta and have a direct stimulant effect on the fetal heart.
175e. False – contraindicated in women on monoamine oxidase inhibitors.

2. Practice MCQs II: Questions

1. **Endoplasmic reticulum (ER)**
   a. The 60S subunit of ribosomes is anchored to ER
   b. Smooth ER is abundantly found in hepatocytes
   c. Rough ER is involved in the synthesis of proteins of the plasma membrane
   d. Smooth ER is responsible for peptide formation
   e. Ribosomes account for the basophilic granularity in rough ER

2. **Mitochondria**
   a. Are 20–50 μm long
   b. Have an outer layer with numerous folds called 'cristae'
   c. Have enzymes for electron transport chain
   d. Have enzymes for citric acid cycle
   e. Their DNA is exclusively of paternal origin

3. **Chromosomes**
   a. Are DNA proteins
   b. Are present in the nucleus
   c. Are outside the nucleus during mitosis
   d. Number in each cell is not species specific
   e. At least one X chromosome is essential for survival

4. **With regard to mitosis**
   a. It is described in four stages
   b. DNA is equally distributed between two daughter cells
   c. The chromatin becomes recognizable as chromosomes during the prophase
   d. The chromatin moves towards the equator of the spindle during the prophase
   e. The division of the cytoplasm begins during the metaphase

5. **The following drugs arrest mitosis in the metaphase**
   a. Colchicine
   b. Podophyllotoxin
   c. Colcemid
   d. Cisapride
   e. Vinblastine

6. **Chorionic villus sampling (CVS)**
   a. Is taking a sample from the amniotic fluid
   b. Is done only by the abdominal route
   c. Is recommended from 9 weeks onwards
   d. Provides a cytogenetic diagnostic result in 99% of the cases
   e. In 1–2% of cases, placental mosaicism is seen

7. The following are correctly matched (haemoglobin and type of globin polypeptide chains)

a. HbA – $\alpha_2\beta_2$
b. HbF – $\alpha_2\delta_2$
c. Gower 1 – $\zeta_2\epsilon_2$
d. HbA_2 – $\alpha_2\gamma_2$
e. Gower II (embryonic) – $\alpha_2\epsilon_2$

8. The following are features of trisomy 18

a. Rocker-bottom feet
b. Wide mouth
c. Large testis
d. Occipital protuberance
e. Low-set eyebrows

9. The following chromosomal aberrations and clinical syndromes are correctly matched:

a. 47XXY – Klinefelter syndrome
b. 45XO/XY – Turner mosaic
c. 45XO – Turner syndrome
d. Trisomy 13 – Down syndrome
e. Trisomy 18 – cri-du-chat syndrome

10. H-Y antigen

a. Is a Y-linked histocompatibility antigen
b. Plays a main role in tissue transplantation
c. Is important for ovarian function
d. Is important for testicular function
e. Is important for testicular differentiation

11. Y-linked inherited conditions include

a. Hairy pinna
b. Partial colour blindness
c. Vitamin D-resistant rickets
d. Haemophilia
e. H-Y antigen

12. Mitochondrial inheritance

a. Leber optic atrophy
b. Angelman syndrome
c. Hereditary blindness
d. Prader–Willi syndrome
e. Muscular dystrophy

13. Phenylketonuria
a. Has an autosomal dominant inheritance pattern
b. Is an example of pleiotropy
c. Causes learning disability
d. Occurs due to deficiency of phenylalanine decarboxylase
e. Causes accumulation of tyrosine in the blood

14. Diseases with deficient DNA repair
a. Xeroderma pigmentosum
b. Bloom syndrome
c. Ataxia telangiectasia
d. Sickle cell anaemia
e. Fanconi anaemia

15. X-linked recessive inheritance
a. Is transmitted from an affected male to half of his grandsons through his daughters
b. Is never transmitted from male to male
c. Is common in females
d. If a carrier female marries a normal male, 50% of the sons would be affected
e. If a carrier female marries an affected male, 50% of the sons would be affected

16. Peroxisomes
a. Are formed in rough endoplasmic reticulum
b. Contain enzymes for the citric acid cycle
c. Contain the enzymes for β-oxidation of fatty acids
d. Produce H_2O_2 for destroying microorganisms
e. Contain the enzyme catalase to detoxify H_2O_2 metabolites

17. Autosomal dominant inheritance
a. The overall prevalence is 1:1000
b. Shows variable expression
c. An allele is expressed in a homozygous state
d. An allele is expressed in a heterozygous state
e. If one parent is heterozygous affected, half the children are affected

18. The conditions that are inherited as autosomal dominant include
a. Phenylketonuria
b. Achondroplasia
c. Porphyria variegata
d. Sickle cell disease
e. Brachydactyly

19. **In autosomal dominant inheritance**
   a. The transmission of the trait is influenced by the sex
   b. The person who is unaffected transmits the trait to their children
   c. The trait appears in every generation
   d. Normally, there is no skipping generation
   e. Males have more chance of getting the trait than females

20. **Examples of non-dysjunction during meiosis include**
   a. Klinefelter syndrome
   b. Turner syndrome
   c. Prader–Willi syndrome
   d. Meigs syndrome
   e. Down syndrome

21. **Robertsonian translocation**
   a. Is named after Robertson
   b. The incidence in humans is 1:1000 births
   c. A carrier is phenotypically abnormal
   d. Usually involves chromosome 15
   e. Is seen in 2% of all cases of Down syndrome

22. **Autosomal recessive inheritance**
   a. The overall prevalence is 10:1000
   b. Is expressed in heterozygous state
   c. Males and females have equal chance of being affected
   d. Usually affected individual has heterozygous parents
   e. More common in children with parents of consanguineous marriage

23. **Granuloma formation is seen in conditions such as**
   a. Actinomycosis
   b. Yaws
   c. Listeriosis
   d. Syphilis
   e. Leprosy

24. **Examples of X-linked recessive conditions include**
   a. Glucose-6-phosphate dehydrogenase
   b. Testicular feminization syndrome
   c. Vitamin D-resistant rickets
   d. Sickle cell disease
   e. Duchenne muscular dystrophy

25. **Examples of X-linked dominant conditions include**
   a. Red–green colour blindness
   b. Vitamin D-resistant rickets
   c. Xg blood group
   d. Hairy ears
   e. Haemophilia

26. **X-linked dominant inheritance**
    a. The trait manifests in the homozygous state
    b. The trait manifests in the heterozygous state
    c. Is twice as common in males as in females
    d. Affected males transmit the trait to their sons
    e. If an affected male marries an affected heterozygous female, all the daughters would be affected

27. **Lysosomes**
    a. Are formed in the smooth endoplasmic reticulum
    b. Mature only in the Golgi apparatus
    c. Secondary lysosomes emerge from the Golgi apparatus
    d. Take part in many metabolic events
    e. Degrade the old cytoplasm

28. **The following organisms cause toxic shock syndrome**
    a. *Staphylococcus aureus*
    b. *Gardnerella vaginalis*
    c. *Streptococcus pyogenes*
    d. *Trichomonas vaginalis*
    e. *Peptostreptococcus species*

29. **The following cells can regenerate**
    a. Epithelium of the gut
    b. Epithelium of the skin
    c. Hepatic cells
    d. Osteocytes
    e. Bone marrow

30. **The following are chemical carcinogens**
    a. Aflatoxins
    b. Nitrosamines
    c. Nitric oxide
    d. Asbestos
    e. Aniline dye

31. **Carcinoid tumour**
    a. Commonest site of origin is the appendix
    b. Is a fast-growing tumour
    c. Is derived from goblet cells in the intestine
    d. Is derived from Kulchitsky cells in the intestine
    e. Cells have a strong affinity for silver stains

32. **Von Willebrand factor (vWf)**
    a. Is produced by endothelial cells
    b. Is produced by megakaryocytes
    c. Is required for platelet adhesion
    d. Decreases the half-life of factor VIII
    e. Increases the half-life of factor VII

33. **Haemoglobin dissociation curve**
   a. Shifts to the right in acidotic conditions
   b. Shifts to the right occur in conditions with low $PaCO_2$ levels
   c. Shift to the right indicates increased affinity of O_2 for haemoglobin
   d. Shift to the right indicates decreased affinity of O_2 for haemoglobin
   e. Bohr effect is seen with a shift to the right of the dissociation curve

34. **With regard to antibody type**
   a. The primary immune response produces IgG
   b. The secondary immune response produces IgM
   c. IgE antibody is found on the surface of mast cells
   d. IgE is the secretory immunoglobulin
   e. IgM antibody crosses the placenta

35. **The following statements are true regarding complement deficiency**
   a. C3 deficiency is associated with recurrent bacterial infections
   b. C1 deficiency is associated with recurrent bacterial infections
   c. C3 deficiency is associated with inefficient phagocytosis
   d. C1 esterase deficiency is associated with hereditary angioneurotic oedema
   e. C2 deficiency is associated with immune complex disease

36. **The type of collagen seen in various organs**
   a. Type I is seen in tendons
   b. Type I is seen in cartilage
   c. Type I is seen in bones
   d. Type IV is exclusively seen in blood vessels
   e. Type III is seen in the uterus

37. **Menstrual cycle and histological changes in the endometrium**
   a. Proliferative phase – highly tortuous glands
   b. Secretory phase – simple tubular glands
   c. Secretory phase – glands are rich in glycogen
   d. Proliferative phase – stroma highly cellular
   e. Secretory phase – stroma highly cellular

38. **Malabsorption is caused by**
   a. Coeliac disease
   b. Tropical sprue
   c. Cystic fibrosis
   d. Whipple disease
   e. Crohn disease

39. **Which dermatological manifestations of systemic disease are paired together correctly?**
    a. Erythema nodosum – acute rheumatic fever
    b. Erythema chronicum migrans – rheumatoid arthritis
    c. Pretibial myxoedema – Graves disease
    d. Hypopigmentation – Addison disease
    e. Hyperpigmentation – hypothyroidism

40. **Hodgkin lymphoma**
    a. Is more common in elderly people
    b. Is more common in young adults
    c. Patients can present with pruritis and fever
    d. Reed–Sternberg cells are seen on histology
    e. Nodular sclerotic type is less common in women

41. **Apoptosis**
    a. Is programmed cell death
    b. Is seen in viral hepatitis
    c. There is synthesis of DNA prior to cell death
    d. There is synthesis of RNA prior to cell death
    e. It involves only single cells

42. **Glycogen**
    a. Liver stores glucose as glycogen
    b. Glycogen from liver is used to maintain blood glucose levels in between meals
    c. Glycogen stores fluctuate during the day
    d. Glycogen in the liver supplies energy for muscle contraction during exercise
    e. Glycogen is the first resource for metabolism in starvation

43. **With regard to types of collagen**
    a. Type 2 is found in bones
    b. Type 2 is found in cartilage
    c. Type 1 is found in skin
    d. Type 7 is found in fetal tissue
    e. Type 1 is found in ligaments

44. **A high carbohydrate meal**
    a. Stimulates release of insulin
    b. Stimulates release of glucagon
    c. Inhibits release of glucagon
    d. Stimulates secretion of growth hormone
    e. Inhibits secretion of growth hormone

45. Adenosine triphosphate (ATP)
a. Is required for protein synthesis
b. Its normal source is carbohydrates
c. Its normal source is fatty acids
d. Its normal source is amino acids
e. Is produced by oxidative phosphorylation

46. Acetyl-CoA
a. Is produced from metabolism of amino acids
b. Is produced from metabolism of fatty acids
c. Enters the glycolytic cycle
d. Enters the citric acid cycle
e. Is converted to 10 molecules of CO_2 and 24 atoms of hydrogen

47. With regard to glycolysis
a. The enzymes responsible for this are in the nucleus
b. The enzymes responsible for this are in the cytoplasm
c. Conversion of glucose to glucose 6-phosphate is the first step in the pathway
d. One molecule of glucose is converted to three molecules of pyruvic acid
e. Conversion of glucose to glucose 6-phosphate is energy dependent

48. During the glycolytic pathway
a. Conversion of fructose 6-phosphate to fructose 1,6-diphosphate is energy dependent
b. Conversion of glucose 6-phosphate to fructose 6-phosphate is energy dependent
c. Conversion of 1,3-diphosphate to 3-phosphoglycerate is energy dependent
d. Conversion of phosphoenolpyruvate to pyruvate is energy dependent
e. Conversion of glucose to glucose 6-phosphate is energy dependent

49. The reaction catalysed by phosphofructokinase in glycolytic pathway
a. Is activated by AMP
b. Is activated by citrate
c. Is activated by ATP
d. Is activated by glucose
e. Is activated by fructose 2,6-diphosphate

50. Nicotinamide adenine dinucleotide (NAD^+)
a. Contains positive charge
b. Contains negative charge
c. Hydrogen atom is part of the NAD molecule
d. Proton is released when hydrogen atom is transferred to NAD^+
e. Is involved in various metabolic steps of the citric acid cycle

51. **NADH**
    a. Contains low intrinsic energy
    b. Requires oxygen to provide energy in the form of ATP
    c. Is produced by conversion of malic acid to oxaloacetate in the citric acid cycle
    d. Two molecules of NADH produce six molecules of ATP from ADP
    e. One molecule of NADH produces three molecules of ATP from ADP

52. **Pyruvate**
    a. Is the end-product of aerobic glycolysis
    b. Is the end-product of anaerobic glycolysis
    c. Is transported to mitochondria in order to enter the citric acid cycle
    d. Is converted to acetyl-CoA by the pyruvate dehydrogenase complex
    e. Conversion of phosphoenolpyruvate to pyruvate is the final step in the glycolytic pathway

53. **With regard to pyruvate kinase**
    a. Is activated by fructose 6-phosphate
    b. Is needed for conversion of pyruvate to phosphoenolpyruvate
    c. Is needed in the final step in the glycolytic pathway
    d. Is activated by insulin
    e. Is activated by glucagon

54. **Pyruvate kinase deficiency**
    a. Can cause lymphopenia
    b. Is restricted to white blood cells
    c. Is restricted to red blood cells
    d. Can cause mild, chronic, haemolytic anaemia
    e. Can cause severe, chronic, haemolytic anaemia

55. **Haemoglobin**
    a. Is composed of two globin chains and three haem rings
    b. Haem ring in haemoglobin is synthesized in the cytoplasm
    c. Haem ring in haemoglobin is synthesized in the nucleus
    d. Iron supply is never a rate-limiting step in haem synthesis
    e. Globin synthesis proceeds only in the presence of sufficient haem

56. **Pyruvate dehydrogenase complex**
    a. Decarboxylates pyruvate to acetyl-CoA
    b. Requires five coenzymes
    c. Deficiency is an X-linked recessive condition
    d. Deficiency causes psychomotor retardation
    e. Is inactivated by arsenic poisoning

57. **With regard to glucose metabolism (aerobic and anaerobic)**
   a. Aerobic metabolism produces 38 ATP (malate–aspartate shuttle) per glucose molecule
   b. Aerobic metabolism produces 40 ATP (glycerol 3-phosphate or G3P shuttle) per glucose molecule
   c. Anaerobic metabolism produces 10 ATP per glucose molecule
   d. Aerobic metabolism produces 36 ATP (G3P shuttle) per glucose molecule
   e. Anaerobic metabolism produces 2 ATP per glucose molecule

58. **Adenosine cyclic monophosphate (cAMP)**
   a. Is synthesized from guanosine triphosphate (GTP)
   b. Is activated by protein kinase A
   c. Is slowly degraded by cAMP phosphodiesterases
   d. Is rapidly degraded by cAMP phosphodiesterases
   e. Requires adenylyl cyclase for its synthesis

59. **Factors causing K^+ to move out of the cell include**
   a. Hyperinsulinaemia
   b. Hypothyroidism
   c. Alkalosis
   d. Acidosis
   e. Severe cell damage

60. **During prolonged fasting**
   a. The brain uses more ketones than glucose
   b. There is decreased gluconeogenesis in the liver
   c. Fatty acid oxidation is increased in the muscles
   d. Ketone use is increased in the muscles
   e. Ketone use is decreased in the muscles

61. **With regard to prostaglandin synthesis**
   a. It is derived from arachidonic acid
   b. It is synthesized from 20-carbon fatty acid chains
   c. Membrane phospholipids are the source of arachidonic acid
   d. Cyclooxygenase converts PGE_2 to PGH_2
   e. Isomerases convert PGH_2 to $PGF_{2\alpha}$ and PGE_2

62. **Nitric oxide**
   a. Is produced from methionine
   b. Has a half-life of 5 minutes
   c. Is released by the endothelial cells of the blood vessels
   d. Mediates vasoconstriction during pregnancy
   e. Mediates vasodilatation during pregnancy

63. **With regard to urea and the urea cycle in humans**
    a. Amino acid detoxification begins only during the urea cycle
    b. Amino acid detoxification begins before the urea cycle
    c. Glutamate is oxidatively deaminated to ammonia
    d. The final reaction in the urea cycle requires arginase
    e. Most of the amino acid detoxification occurs in the kidney

64. **During catecholamine synthesis**
    a. Tyrosine is converted to 3,4-dihydroxyphenylalanine (dopa)
    b. Tyrosine hydroxylase converts phenylalanine to tyrosine
    c. Tyrosine hydroxylase is required to convert tyrosine to dopa
    d. Dopa is converted to dopamine by dopa decarboxylase
    e. Dopamine is decarboxylated to noradrenaline

65. **Fats**
    a. Contain more oxygen than carbohydrates
    b. Contain less oxygen than proteins
    c. Are composed of triacylglycerols
    d. Yield less energy on oxidation than from an equivalent amount of carbohydrates
    e. One gram of fat yields 7 kcal of energy

66. **Cervical intraepithelial neoplasia (CIN)**
    a. Is a cytological diagnosis
    b. Is characterized by large abnormal nuclei and reduced cytoplasm
    c. Immature cells are present in the upper third of the epithelium in CIN1
    d. Immature cells are present in the lower and middle third of the epithelium in CIN2
    e. Immature cells are present in the lower third of the epithelium in CIN3

67. **The transformation zone in the cervix**
    a. Is where the squamous and columnar epithelium meet after puberty
    b. Is where native squamous epithelium changes to columnar epithelium
    c. Is where most precancerous changes occur
    d. Contains cervical crypt openings
    e. Nabothian cysts can be seen in this area

68. **Squamous metaplasia in the cervix**
    a. Is a physiological process
    b. Always occurs before puberty
    c. Is preceded by reserve cell hyperplasia
    d. Converts squamous to columnar epithelium
    e. Is caused by herpes simplex virus

69. **Referral criteria for colposcopy in the UK include**
   a. Ectropion on speculum examination
   b. Suspicious-looking cervix on speculum examination
   c. One report of mild dyskaryosis
   d. One report of severe dyskaryosis
   e. One report of glandular neoplasia

70. **Acetowhite epithelium may be found in association with**
   a. Cervical intraepithelial neoplasia
   b. Vaginal intraepithelial neoplasia
   c. Human papillomavirus infection
   d. Immature squamous metaplasia
   e. Congenital transformation zone

71. **Fluorescence *in situ* hybridization (FISH)**
   a. Provides information about specific chromosomes studied
   b. Provides information about the complete karyotype
   c. Is used for detection of chromosomal microdeletion syndromes
   d. Can be performed on metaphase chromosomal preparations of cultured lymphocytes
   e. Can be performed on interphase nuclei from chorionic villi

72. **Examples of microdeletion syndromes**
   a. Prader–Willi syndrome
   b. Fragile X syndrome
   c. Angelman syndrome
   d. DiGeorge syndrome
   e. Kartagener syndrome

73. **Innate or non-specific immunity**
   a. Is antigen specific
   b. Is not antigen specific
   c. Response is not antigen dependent
   d. Response is antigen dependent
   e. Lag period is present between exposure and response

74. **Natural killer cells**
   a. Resemble neutrophils in their morphology
   b. Are slightly larger than lymphocytes
   c. Are identified by the presence of CD3 cell surface marker
   d. Are identified by the presence of CD56 and CD16 cell surface markers
   e. Are capable of killing virus-infected cells

75. Immunoglobulins
  a. Are serum proteins acting as antigens
  b. Are made of four polypeptide chains
  c. Light chains differ in each immunoglobulin
  d. Heavy chains are alike in all classes of immunoglobulins
  e. Contain a variable region and a constant region

76. The following terminologies indicate tissue necrosis
  a. Surgical amputation
  b. Postmortem examination
  c. Autolysis
  d. Gangrene
  e. Caseation

77. Complement
  a. Is a protein
  b. Is required for lysis of an antigen-bearing cell
  c. Is active in the destruction of microorganisms
  d. Protects against rejection of implanted tissue
  e. Brings about destruction of antigen-bearing cells by facilitating phagocytosis

78. Graft rejection
  a. Is an immune response
  b. Antigen similarity increases the chance of rejection
  c. 'T'-effector lymphocyte reacts with the graft tissue leading to rejection
  d. Homograft rejection occurs in identical twins
  e. Homograft rejection occurs in non-identical twins where mixing of the placental circulation has taken place *in utero*

79. The following terminologies about graft are correctly matched
  a. Autograft – is a tissue graft from the host's own tissues
  b. Isograft – is a tissue graft from a donor to a host with different genotypes
  c. Allograft – is a tissue graft from a donor to a host having the same genotype
  d. Xenograft – is a tissue graft between members of different species
  e. Homograft – is a tissue graft from a donor to a host with identical genotype

80. The human major histocompatibility complex (MHC)
  a. Is divided into five classes
  b. Lies on the short arm of chromosome 6
  c. Class I molecules are responsible for transplant rejection
  d. Class II region codes for complement protein
  e. Class III molecules are present on the surface of B cells

81. With regard to the human major histocompatibility complex (MHC)
   a. It contains genes that control antigens which influence allograft rejection
   b. Class I molecules are expressed on all nucleated cells
   c. Type 1 diabetes mellitus occurs at a higher frequency in individuals with the DR3/-4 haplotype
   d. Class I molecules are expressed on human red blood cells
   e. The genes of the MHC are equally inherited from each parent

82. The following statements about vaccines are true
   a. *Haemophilus influenzae* type b vaccine is 95% effective
   b. BCG (Bacille Calmette–Guérin) prevents pulmonary tuberculosis
   c. MMR (measles, mumps and rubella) vaccine is a live attenuated vaccine
   d. Hepatitis B vaccine is a live attenuated vaccine
   e. Vaccine against human papillomavirus (HPV) is a subunit vaccine, composed of capsid protein

83. Vaccines that should be avoided in the immunocompromised patient include
   a. Yellow fever
   b. Hepatitis A
   c. *Haemophilus influenzae* type b
   d. Rabies
   e. Japanese encephalitis

84. Haemolytic disease of the newborn
   a. Is associated with a positive direct Coombs test in the cord blood
   b. Is associated with an increased prothrombin time
   c. Is associated with jaundice after 24 hours
   d. Is associated with jaundice at birth
   e. Is characterized by the absence of erythroblasts in cord blood

85. Sex differentiation
   a. Sex-determining region on Y chromosome (SRY gene) is responsible for the differentiation of the gonad to become a testis
   b. Individual with 46XY and a mutation with SRY gene will develop ovaries
   c. The absence of Y chromosomes will promote an embryo to develop into a male
   d. The presence of three X chromosomes and one Y chromosome will lead to maleness
   e. The presence of five X chromosomes and one Y chromosome will lead to femaleness

86. Dihydrotestosterone (DHT)
a. Is derived from dehydroepiandrosterone
b. Formation depends on the presence of an aromatase enzyme
c. Brings about the development of external genitalia in the male during intrauterine life
d. Deficiency of the enzyme required for its formation results in the development of male internal genitalia (testis)
e. Deficiency of the enzyme required for its formation results in the development of female external genitalia

87. Genetic basis of hydatidiform mole
a. Triploidy is seen in a partial mole
b. Chromosomes are solely of maternal origin in a partial mole
c. Fertilization of an ovum by two sperm results in a complete mole
d. A partial mole occurs by fertilization of an empty ovum by two sperm
e. Chromosomes are purely of paternal origin in a complete mole

88. Sex chromatin
a. Is derived from the Y chromosome
b. Stains lightly with basic dyes
c. Is seen in the metaphase cells
d. Is seen in the interphase cells
e. Is also called the Barr body

89. Lyon hypothesis (the principle of X chromosome inactivation)
a. Only one X chromosome is active in the somatic cells of mammals
b. Inactivation of X chromosomes occurs in adult life
c. Inactivated X chromosome is mainly of paternal origin
d. Inactivated X chromosome is mainly of maternal origin
e. Males do not have a sex chromatin or Barr body

90. During anaphase of mitosis
a. Chromosomes move towards the equator of the spindle
b. Cytoplasmic division begins by infolding of the cell at the equator
c. Two new chromosomes move apart, one towards each pole of the cell
d. Nucleoli disintegrate and disappear
e. The nuclear membrane reappears

91. A mutational change in gene can be induced by
a. X-rays
b. Mustard gas
c. Nitrous acid
d. Formaldehyde
e. Gamma rays from radium

92. **The presence of the following conditions offers resistance or protection against severe malaria**
   a. α-Thalassaemia
   b. Sickle cell trait (HbAS)
   c. G6PD deficiency
   d. FyFy genotype in the Duffy blood group
   e. Sickle cell disease (HbSS)

93. **In a standard 12-lead ECG**
   a. Lead III is the signal between the aVL electrode on the left arm and the aVF electrode on the left leg
   b. Lead aVF has the positive electrode on the left leg. The negative electrode is on the left arm
   c. Lead V1 is placed in the fourth intercostal space (between ribs 4 and 5) to the left of the sternum
   d. A P–R interval of over 100 milliseconds (ms) may indicate a first-degree heart block
   e. The normal electrical axis lies between -30° and $+90^\circ$

94. **In obstetric ultrasound**
   a. The abdominal probe most commonly used operates at a frequency of 6–7.5 MHz
   b. Lateral resolution is mediated by the beam width
   c. Increasing the frequency of the probe increases the field of view
   d. The transvaginal probe typically operates with a higher-frequency probe than the abdominal probe
   e. The wavelength determines the axial resolution

95. **As regards ultrasound and Doppler scanning**
   a. Continuous-wave Doppler scanning is more commonly used in obstetrics than pulsed-wave Doppler scanning
   b. Red colour denotes flow away from the transducer and blue colour denotes flow towards the transducer in colour Doppler imaging
   c. Aliasing is a technical artefact seen during use of pulsed-wave Doppler scanning
   d. Doppler frequency is determined only by angle of insonation
   e. MI (mechanical Index), TIS (soft-tissue thermal index) and TIB (thermal index for bone) indicate safety indices in the use of Doppler scanning

96. **In urodynamics**
   a. The rectal pressure probe measures the intra-abdominal pressure
   b. The bladder pressure probe measures the intravesical pressure
   c. Free uroflowmetry measures how fast the patient can empty their bladder
   d. A cough or Valsalva manouvre can be performed to confirm genuine stress incontinence
   e. Cystometry alone can demonstrate the reasons for voiding difficulties

97. Electrosurgery
  a. For the safe use of bipolar diathermy a split return electrode is required
  b. Skin burns are more common with unipolar diathermy
  c. Options to cut, coagulate, desiccate or fulgurate rely on changes in power and the electrical waveform
  d. To minimize the effects of muscle and neural stimulation, a return pad is used for unipolar diathermy
  e. With unipolar diathermy the electric current preferentially runs through the blood vessels

98. In radiotherapy
  a. β-Rays are composed of electrons
  b. Intracavitary radiotherapy (brachytherapy) works by the release of particles that have high penetrating power
  c. Necrosis within tumours reduces sensitivity to radiotherapy
  d. Less differentiated tumours are more sensitive to radiotherapy
  e. Squamous cell carcinoma of the cervix is generally less sensitive to radiotherapy than adenocarcinoma of the cervix

99. Imaging
  a. The dose of radiation used in an abdominal CT is approximately ten times the dose of a plain chest radiograph
  b. No effects of MRI on the fetus have been demonstrated
  c. Ventilation–perfusion scan ($\dot{V}/\dot{Q}$ scan) performed during pregnancy has less risk to the fetus than CT pulmonary angiogram in the diagnosis of a pulmonary embolus
  d. $\dot{V}/\dot{Q}$ scan performed during pregnancy has less risk to the mother than CT pulmonary angiogram in the diagnosis of a pulmonary embolus
  e. MRI has less movement artefact than CT

100. The risks involved in amniocentesis include
  a. Fetal puncture
  b. Amnionitis
  c. Amniotic fluid leakage
  d. Amniotic fluid embolism
  e. Miscarriage

101. Chorionic villus biopsy (CVS)
  a. Is associated with limb defect when performed after 9 weeks
  b. Is associated with miscarriage in 1–2% of the cases
  c. Is used as a screening test for Down syndrome
  d. Is associated with vaginal bleeding
  e. Is always done under ultrasound guidance

102. The uses of ultrasound examination during the first trimester of pregnancy include

a. Measurement of the crown–rump length to determine exact gestational age
b. Measurement of the biparietal diameter to determine exact gestational age
c. Measurement of the femur length to determine exact gestational age
d. Detection of gross fetal malformations, e.g. anencephaly
e. Perform nuchal translucency scan to determine risk of Down syndrome

103. The following abnormalities can be detected by ultrasonography

a. Duodenal atresia
b. Diaphragmatic hernia
c. Renal agenesis
d. Encephalocele
e. Omphalocele

104. Clinical syndromes caused by chromosomal (autosomal) aberrations include

a. Cri-du-chat syndrome
b. Turner syndrome
c. Edwards syndrome
d. Klinefelter syndrome
e. Patau syndrome

105. Klinefelter syndrome and cytogenetics

a. Individuals with the condition are phenotypically male and show absence of sex chromatin
b. The error during gametogenesis can occur during the first meiotic division
c. The error during gametogenesis can occur during the second meiotic division
d. The error during gametogenesis is paternal in 90% of the cases
e. Of all patients with this syndrome 80–90% have the karyotype 46XY/47XXY

106. The features of Turner syndrome include

a. Epicanthic folds
b. Coarctation of the aorta
c. High-arched palate
d. Short metatarsals
e. Single palmar crease

107. The following are due to inborn errors of carbohydrate metabolism

a. Pompe disease
b. McArdle disease
c. Lesch–Nyam syndrome
d. Galactosaemia
e. Tay–Sachs disease

108. **Tay–Sachs disease**
   a. Is inherited as an autosomal dominant disease
   b. Is associated with early onset in infancy
   c. Is associated with cherry-red spot on the macula
   d. Is characterized by severe learning disability
   e. Is associated with deficiency of the enzyme sphingomyelinase

109. **Wilson disease**
   a. Is an autosomal dominant condition
   b. Can lead to cirrhosis of liver
   c. Can cause deposition of copper in the basal ganglia
   d. Is associated with an increase in the serum ceruloplasmin levels
   e. Kayser–Fleischer ring is seen in the retina

110. **With regard to sickle cell haemoglobulin (HbS) in RBCs**
   a. Low oxygen tension promotes sickling of these RBCs
   b. High oxygen tension promotes sickling of these RBCs
   c. Acidosis and dehydration promote sickling of these RBCs
   d. HbS is diagnosed by haemoglobin electrophoresis
   e. HbS differs from normal haemoglobin (HbA) in the α-chain component

111. **The following are true with regard to different variants of haemoglobin**
   a. Haemoglobin Bart is made of four β-chains
   b. Haemoglobin H is made of four γ-chains
   c. In haemoglobin C, glutamic acid is replaced by lysine at the sixth amino acid position from the N-terminal end in the α-chain
   d. Haemoglobin S is made of two α- and two β-chains
   e. Haemoglobin A is made of two α- and two β-chains

112. **Thalassaemia**
   a. Is associated with characteristic facies due to hyperplasia of the bone marrow in facial and skull bones
   b. Is associated with accumulation of only β-chains in the red cell precursors
   c. Is associated with accumulation of only α-chains in the red cell precursors
   d. Is associated with hypoplasia of the bone marrow, leading to severe anaemia
   e. Is characterized by target cell appearance of red cells on peripheral blood smear

113. **With respect to ECG changes during pregnancy**
   a. There is a left axis deviation
   b. May show high-voltage QRS complexes
   c. Ventricular systoles are common
   d. May show depression of the ST segment
   e. May show low-voltage QRS complexes

114. Metabolic disorders that can be detected by screening of the newborn include
a. Homocystinuria
b. Phenylketonuria
c. Galactosaemia
d. Cystinuria
e. Histidinaemia

115. The following results of detection tests are correctly matched with X-linked disorders
a. Increased serum creatine kinase – Becker muscular dystrophy
b. Reduced G6PD in erythrocytes – maple syrup disease
c. Reduced serum factor VIII – haemophilia B
d. Increased serum phosphorus – vitamin D-resistant rickets
e. Reduced steroid sulphatase – X-linked ichthyosis

116. Red blood cells
a. Utilize glucose as a fuel
b. Cannot survive without glucose
c. Generate ATP by aerobic glycolysis
d. Generate ATP by anaerobic glycolysis
e. Generate ATP by fatty acid oxidation

117. Calcitonin
a. Is a peptide that binds to osteoclasts
b. Can be given by the oral route
c. Can be given by the nasal route
d. Promotes bone absorption
e. Causes hot flushes and diarrhoea

118. Selective oestrogen receptor modulator (SERM)
a. Reduces the occurrence of vertebral fractures by 30–50%
b. Reduces occurrence of non-vertebral fractures by 50%
c. Decreases the incidence of breast cancer
d. Does not have any effect on endometrium
e. Reduces the risk of coronary heart disease

119. The following antibiotics are correctly matched with their mode of action
a. Clavulanic acid – inhibitor of β-lactamases
b. Gentamicin – damages cytoplasmic membranes
c. Tetracyclines – inhibit translation (protein synthesis)
d. Cephalosporins – inhibit steps in cell wall (peptidoglycan) synthesis
e. Clindamycin – inhibits translation (protein synthesis)

120. The following methods of sterilization are effective for killing bacterial endospores

a. Formaldehyde
b. Boiling
c. Autoclave
d. Pasteurization
e. Irradiation

121. Concerning meticillin-resistant *Staphylococcus aureus* (MRSA) infection

a. Transmission can be prevented by appropriate hand hygiene
b. Community-acquired MRSA strains display enhanced virulence compared with hospital-acquired strains
c. Includes strains of the bacterium that are resistant to meticillin, but sensitive to cephalosporins
d. MRSA and vancomycin-resistant enterococci (VREs) are the most commonly encountered multiple drug-resistant organisms in patients residing in non-hospital health-care facilities
e. MRSA is sensitive to vancomycin and fusidic acid

122. Concerning hepatitis B virus (HBV) infection

a. HBV surface antigen is detectable in the bloodstream 3–5 days after infection
b. The presence of HBV surface and envelope antigens in the blood may indicate chronic infection
c. The presence of HBV surface antigen is the best marker for infectivity
d. The antibody to HBV core antigen is the first antibody to appear
e. The presence of antibody to the HBV envelope antigen (HBeAg) increases the risk of transmission to the fetus

123. The following are important in the principles of DNA cloning

a. Isolation of DNA sequence of interest
b. Obtaining multiples of RNA from DNA
c. Obtaining multiples of DNA from an organism such as a bacterium
d. Isolation of pure DNA in large quantities
e. Isolation of pure RNA from DNA

124. The following are used as vectors in the DNA-cloning process

a. Cosmids
b. Bacteriophages
c. Plasmids
d. Nucleocapsid
e. Yeast artificial chromosomes

125. **With regard to the polymerase chain reaction (PCR)**
   a. It is an artificial means of replicating short DNA sequences quickly
   b. DNA polymerase is required for DNA replication
   c. Only a small quantity of DNA sequence of interest is enough to produce millions of copies
   d. It gives large quantities of impure DNA
   e. The first step in the PCR process is denaturation of the genomic DNA by heating at a high temperature to form single-stranded DNA

126. **The following are true of ribonucleic acid (RNA)**
   a. It is composed of two polynucleotide chains
   b. It is synthesized on a DNA template by transcription
   c. RNA polymerase enzyme is required for transcription
   d. Messenger RNA (mRNA) is produced in the cytoplasm
   e. Messenger RNA and transfer RNA (tRNA) are both involved in protein synthesis

127. **NHS cervical cancer screening:**
   a. Women aged 20–64 should be screened every 2 years
   b. Women aged 25–49 should be screened every 3 years
   c. Women aged 50–64 should be screened every 5 years
   d. Women under the age of 25 should not be screened unless already included in the screening programme
   e. Women over the age of 65 should be screened only if they have not been screened since the age of 50

128. **With regard to human papillomavirus**
   a. HPV type depends on RNA homology
   b. Polymerase chain reaction (PCR) is used for its diagnosis
   c. HPV6 and -11 cause genital warts
   d. HPV33 and -35 are oncogenic
   e. HPV16 and -18 cause most cases of cervical cancer

129. **Severe dyskaryosis**
   a. Is caused by exposure to human papillomavirus
   b. Is characterized by large hyperchromatic nuclei on cytology
   c. Is characterized by pyknotic nuclei
   d. Is best treated by radical trachelectomy
   e. Is best treated by total hysterectomy

130. **The following are advantages of liquid-based cytology (LBC)**
   a. It dramatically increases the number of inadequate smears
   b. It reduces the workload for primary care trusts
   c. It reduces the workload for cytology laboratories
   d. The same sample can be used for chlamydia testing
   e. The same sample can be used for testing HPV

131. Indications for knife cone cervical biopsy
- a. Cervical intraepithelial neoplasia I (CIN I)
- b. Cervical intraepithelial neoplasia II (CIN II)
- c. Satisfactory colposcopy with HPV changes
- d. Suspicion of a glandular lesion
- e. Microinvasive disease

132. Complications of the knife cone cervical biopsy procedure include
- a. Secondary haemorrhage
- b. Premature rupture of the membranes
- c. Infection
- d. Preterm delivery
- e. Pre-eclampsia

133. Routine antenatal booking investigations in low-risk women include
- a. ELISA test for hepatitis B
- b. Blood group and antibody levels
- c. Biophysical profile
- d. Cordocentesis
- e. Fetal echocardiogram

134. With regard to antepartum haemorrhage (APH)
- a. It is per vaginal bleeding after 24 weeks of pregnancy but before delivery of the baby
- b. Abruption is the cause when per vaginal bleeding occurs before 24 weeks of pregnancy
- c. Cervical cancer could be a cause of APH
- d. Vasa praevia is one of the recognized causes of APH
- e. Anti-D should be given to all women presenting with APH

135. Pre-eclampsia
- a. Is synonymous with proteinuric pregnancy-induced hypertension
- b. Is due to inadequate invasion of the trophoblasts into the spiral arteries
- c. Is associated with fetal macrosomia
- d. Is associated with hydrops fetalis
- e. Is associated with systemic lupus erythematosus (SLE)

136. The findings on obstetric ultrasound scan in fetuses with IUGR due to placental insufficiency include
- a. Increased liquor volume
- b. Increased weight of the baby
- c. Increased resistance index in the umbilical artery
- d. Absent end-diastolic flow
- e. Reversal of end-diastolic flow

137. **The following are components of the Bishop score**
   a. Uterocervical length
   b. Cervical dilatation
   c. Position of the uterus
   d. Consistency of the cervix
   e. Station of the presenting part in relation to ischial tuberosity

138. **The following fetal and placental factors are proposed for onset of labour**
   a. Maturation of the fetal hypothalamic–pituitary–adrenal axis
   b. Secretion of adrenocorticotrophic hormone (ACTH) by the fetal pituitary
   c. Secretion of cortisol by the fetal adrenal gland in response to ACTH
   d. Secretion of corticotrophin-releasing hormone (CRH) by the placenta, resulting in stimulation of the fetal adrenal gland
   e. Secretion of the hormone progesterone by the placenta

139. **With regard to oxytocin receptors in the uterus**
   a. The majority of these receptors are in the upper uterine segment
   b. They form the link between oxytocin in the fetal circulation and the myometrial cells
   c. The sensitivity of the myometrial cells is dependent on the receptor density rather than on just the increased output of oxytocin
   d. The sensitivity of the myometrial cells is dependent on the increased output of oxytocin rather than on oxytocin receptors
   e. Increased concentration of progesterone promotes formation of the oxytocin receptors

140. **Physiology of myometrial contraction**
   a. Oxytocin is responsible for the release of calcium in myometrial cells
   b. The interaction between actin and myosin is triggered by the release of calcium
   c. The interaction between actin and myosin promotes production of the energy (ATP) required to initiate uterine contraction
   d. The contractions are stronger in the lower segment than in the upper segment
   e. The contractions are initiated at the cornua of the uterus and are strongest in the upper segment

141. **Oxytocin**
   a. Is produced in the hypothalamus
   b. Is stored in the anterior lobe of the pituitary gland until required
   c. Acts as a hormone as well as a neurotransmitter
   d. Is secreted continuously from the pituitary in late pregnancy
   e. Secretion is increased by the Ferguson reflex in labour

142. Polycystic ovarian syndrome (PCOS) is associated with
a. Insulin resistance
b. Increase in serum testosterone
c. Irregular menstrual cycles
d. Type 1 diabetes mellitus
e. Increase in sex hormone-binding globulin (SHBG)

143. In the UK, the following statements are true with regard to heavy menstrual bleeding (menorrhagia)
a. Ninety per cent of women receive medical treatment before referral to a specialist by a GP
b. One in 20 women aged 30–49 consults a GP for menorrhagia
c. It is the main presenting problem in at least 80% of those who go on to have a hysterectomy
d. At least half of all women who have a hysterectomy for menorrhagia have a normal uterus
e. According to NICE guidelines, menorrhagia is defined as excessive menstrual loss that interferes with the quality of life

144. The following are recognized treatments of menorrhagia due to dysfunctional uterine bleeding (DUB)
a. Tranexamic acid
b. Myomectomy
c. Uterine artery embolization
d. Endometrial ablative procedures
e. Mirena intrauterine system (IUS)

145. The causes of menorrhagia include
a. Adenomyosis
b. Copper intrauterine contraceptive device (IUD)
c. Hyperthyroidism
d. Von Willebrand factor deficiency
e. Subserous fibroids

146. The causes of thrombocytopenia in pregnancy include
a. Systemic lupus erythematosus
b. Haemolytic–uraemic syndrome
c. HELLP syndrome
d. Disseminated intravascular coagulation
e. Haemophilia

147. The laboratory diagnosis of disseminated intravascular coagulation (DIC) is made by findings of
a. Decrease in fibrinogen
b. Decrease in fibrin degradation products (FDPs)
c. Increase in thrombin time (TT)
d. Decrease in prothrombin time (PT)
e. Increase in activated partial thromboplastin time (APTT)

148. In von Willebrand disease
a. Factor IX is reduced
b. Clotting time is prolonged
c. Bleeding time is prolonged
d. APTT may be prolonged
e. Factor VIII levels fall rapidly during the postpartum period

149. Thrombotic thrombocytopenic purpura is characterized by
a. Aplastic anaemia
b. Microangiopathic haemolytic anaemia
c. Neurological symptoms
d. Hypertension
e. Thrombocytopenia

150. Malaria in pregnancy
a. Can be caused by *Plasmodium falciparum*
b. Can be caused by *Plasmodium vivax*
c. Decreases the risk of premature labour
d. Increases the birth weight of the baby
e. Can result in congenital malaria by transplacental spread

151. Hyperemesis gravidarum
a. Is a diagnosis of exclusion
b. Is associated with deranged renal function tests
c. May be associated with abnormal thyroid function tests
d. Can lead to Mallory–Weiss tear in cases of prolonged vomiting
e. Can be associated with Wernicke encephalopathy in severe cases

152. The following are physiological changes that occur during pregnancy
a. Increase in oxygen consumption by 20%
b. Increase in metabolic rate by 50%
c. Decrease in functional residual capacity due to diaphragmatic elevation in late pregnancy
d. Increase in resting minute ventilation by 40–50%
e. There is rise in arterial PCO_2 and fall in arterial PO_2

153. Risk factors for venous thromboembolism during pregnancy include
a. Paraplegia
b. Sickle cell disease
c. Antithrombin III deficiency
d. Long-haul travel
e. Body mass index (BMI) more than 30

154. In women with pulmonary thromboembolism (PTE), a chest radiograph may show the following findings
a. Wedge-shaped infarction
b. Atelectasis
c. Pericardial effusion
d. Cardiomegaly
e. Areas of translucency in under-perfused lung

155. The imaging studies that are used to make a diagnosis of pulmonary embolism during pregnancy include
a. Ventilation–perfusion scan
b. Computed tomography (CT) scan of the abdomen
c. CT pulmonary angiography (CTPA)
d. Venogram of both legs
e. Duplex Doppler ultrasound scans of femoral and iliac vessels

156. The following statements are true with regard to antibodies in systemic lupus erythematosus (SLE)
a. The most common autoantibody is anti-Rho antibody
b. Antibodies against double-stranded DNA and anti-Smith (anti-Sm) antibody are non-specific antibodies
c. Anti-Rho and anti-La antibodies do not cross the placenta
d. Glomerulonephritis occurs less frequently in women with antibodies to double-stranded DNA
e. Antinuclear antibody is seen in only 50% of the cases

157. The causes of seizures in pregnancy include
a. Thrombotic thrombocytopenic purpura
b. Intracerebral haemorrhage
c. Cerebral vein thrombosis
d. Withdrawal of recreational drugs
e. Eclampsia

158. Myasthenia gravis
a. Is caused by IgM antibodies directed against the nicotinic acetylcholine receptor on the motor end-plate
b. Is associated with weakness and fatigue of smooth muscle
c. Is associated with diplopia and ptosis of the eyelid
d. May rarely cause arthrogryposis multiplex congenita in fetus
e. Diagnosis is made by administration of suxamethonium

159. Pemphigoid gestationis
a. Is an autoimmune disease
b. Is common during pregnancy
c. Is a self-limiting condition
d. Usually occurs in the third trimester
e. Is associated with lesions around the umbilicus, unlike polymorphic eruption of pregnancy

160. The following are causes of acute renal failure during pregnancy
  a. Acute fatty liver of pregnancy
  b. HELLP syndrome
  c. Haemolytic–uraemic syndrome
  d. Massive abruption
  e. Puerperal sepsis

161. With regard to primary maternal cytomegalovirus (CMV) infection
  a. Most women are usually symptomatic
  b. It occurs in 10–20% of pregnant women
  c. The vertical transmission rate to the fetus is around 40%
  d. The fetal damage occurs in 90% of infected fetuses
  e. Recurrent CMV is always associated with fetal damage

162. The following viral infections are associated with high maternal mortality in pregnant women
  a. Hepatitis A
  b. Hepatitis B
  c. Hepatitis E
  d. Varicella-zoster
  e. Japanese B encephalitis

163. The following are true regarding maternal hepatitis C infection
  a. Caesarean section prevents the risk of transmission to the fetus
  b. Caesarean section reduces the risk of transmission to the fetus
  c. Caesarean section increases the risk of transmission to the fetus
  d. If acute maternal infection occurs in the third trimester, infection is not transmitted to the fetus
  e. If the mother is positive for hepatitis C viral RNA, the risk of neonatal infection is around 5–10%

164. With regard to *Listeria monocytogenes*
  a. It is a motile Gram-negative rod
  b. It can multiply at low temperatures
  c. It can cause meningitis in adults
  d. Of the healthy population 90% carry this organism in their bowel
  e. Histological examination of the placenta shows miliary granulomas and necrosis, when infection occurs during pregnancy

165. Mumps
  a. Is an adenovirus
  b. Is highly infectious
  c. Has an incubation period of 7 days
  d. Manifests mainly as meningitis
  e. Can be prevented by vaccination

166. Fetal stem cells
a. Can be obtained from fetal placenta
b. Can be obtained from fetal umbilical cord blood
c. Can be obtained from fetal bone marrow
d. Can be obtained from fetal liver
e. Can be obtained from fetal neural tissue

167. The following are advantages of cord (umbilical) blood banking
a. Cord blood is a rich source of haematopoietic stem cells
b. Cord blood requires stricter criteria for tissue type matching between potential recipient and donor than required for bone marrow donors
c. Cord blood recipients have more severe graft-versus-host disease than bone marrow recipients
d. Cord blood can be used for bone marrow disorders such as leukaemia
e. Cord blood can be used in metabolic disorders such as Hurler syndrome

168. With regard to the amniotic fluid during the second half of pregnancy
a. Most of the fluid is obtained from active sodium and potassium transport across the amniotic membrane
b. Most of the fluid is obtained from active sodium and potassium transport across fetal skin
c. Only a minor amount is obtained from the respiratory tract
d. Most of the fluid is obtained from the gastrointestinal tract
e. Only a minor amount is obtained from fetal micturition

169. Active management of the third stage of labour is associated with
a. Increase in the duration of the third stage of labour
b. Decrease in the duration of the third stage of labour
c. Increase in the proportion of women with blood loss of 500 mL or more
d. Decrease in the proportion of women with nausea and vomiting
e. Increase in the proportion of women with nausea and vomiting

170. Antiphospholipid antibody syndrome (APS) during pregnancy
a. Is associated with recurrent early pregnancy loss
b. Can be associated with thrombotic events or a past history of thromboembolism
c. Is diagnosed by a blood test showing moderate-to-high titres of IgG anticardiolipin antibodies
d. Is associated with abnormal placental function, resulting in fetal loss
e. May be associated with placental changes of infarction, necrosis and thrombosis in women with fetal loss

171. **Which terminologies used in evaluating the safety of heath care and their definitions are matched correctly?**
   a. Medical error – an injury caused by medical management and not by the underlying condition or disease
   b. Near miss – a medical error that does not result in an injury
   c. Adverse event – the use of the wrong management plan to achieve an aim or failure of an action to be completed as intended
   d. Preventable adverse event – an adverse event caused by medical error
   e. Serious untoward incident – an incident occurring within health service premises or in relation to the health service provided, resulting in serious injury to the staff or public or causing major permanent harm or an unexpected death of a patient

172. **The following are the pillars of clinical governance**
   a. Clinical audit
   b. Risk management
   c. Education and training
   d. Clinical effectiveness and research
   e. Patient and public involvement

173. **With regard to the principles of the risk management process**
   a. It is a process meant to improve patient safety and outcome
   b. It involves strategies to optimize the outcome of patient care
   c. It involves strategies to prevent or decrease risks that can lead to potential harm to health and safety of patients
   d. The first step in the risk management process is risk identification
   e. Risk or incident reporting and monitoring of reporting also form part of the risk management process

174. **Clinical Negligence Scheme for Trusts (CNST)**
   a. Is a management programme started in 1990
   b. Provides indemnity cover for NHS bodies in England
   c. Is administered by the NHS litigation authority (NHSLA)
   d. Provides NHS trusts with a set of risk management standards for maternity services
   e. Contributions are significantly lower than the equivalent commercial premiums

175. **With regard to pituitary prolactinomas**
   a. Prolactinomas account for nearly 30% of the pituitary adenomas causing tumoral hyperprolactinaemia
   b. Pituitary microadenomas are found in 10–20% of the normal population as per autopsy studies
   c. Microprolactinomas are typically associated with prolactin values >5000 mU/L
   d. Macroprolactinomas can cause visual field defect and cranial nerve palsies
   e. Surgical treatment is the first-line management in cases of microprolactinomas

2. Practice MCQs II: Answers

1a. True
1b. True
1c. True
1d. False
1e. True

Note
Endoplasmic reticulum (ER) is of two types: (1) smooth ER, (2) rough ER. Rough ER is studded with ribosomes, which account for the basophilic granularity, and is responsible for peptide formation. Smooth ER is responsible for metabolism of small molecules, e.g. detoxification of drugs and poisons. They are present abundantly in hepatocytes where they also help in the synthesis of cholesterol and bile acid. Rough ER helps in the production of hormones and enzymes to be secreted outside the cell, as well as lysosomal enzymes for the digestion of phagocytosed particles.

2a. False – they are 2–5 μm long.
2b. False – the inner layer has numerous folds called cristae.
2c. True
2d. True – the enzymes of the citric acid cycle are present in the mitochondrial matrix. The other functions include oxidation of pyruvate and fatty acids.
2e. False – it is exclusively maternal in origin. It is similar to prokaryotic nucleic acids.

3a. True
3b. True
3c. True
3d. False – the number in each cell is species specific.
3e. True

Note
The vehicles of heredity are chromosomes and it is through fertilization that they are passed on to the next generation. The number of chromosomes in each cell is species specific. The human sperm and ovum each contain half the number of species-specific chromosomes and are therefore called haploid (23 chromosomes). There are two sex chromosomes (X and Y) and 22 pairs of autosomes. Maleness is determined by the Y chromosome. One of the X chromosomes in females is inactive in each cell (Lyon hypothesis) and is present as a clump of chromatin in female nuclei.

4a. True
4b. True
4c. True
4d. False – it occurs during metaphase.
4e. False – it occurs during anaphase.

Note
Mitosis occurs in somatic cells. It is divided into four stages: prophase, metaphase, anaphase and telophase.

During prophase, the chromatin swells up and becomes shorter, to be identified as chromosomes. The nucleoli disappear together with disappearance of the nuclear membrane. Microtubules are synthesized.

During metaphase, the microtubules come to the centre of the cell and chromosomes move to the equator of the spindle.

During anaphase, the chromosomes become grouped at the end of each cell and both groups are diploid. The cytoplasm division begins only in anaphase.

During telophase, the nuclear membrane and nucleoli reappear, the cell divides and each cell has a nucleus in it. The spindle disappears.

5a. True
5b. True
5c. True
5d. False
5e. True

Note
Drugs that bind to tubulin mainly inhibit mitosis by depolymerization of the microtubules. Both podophyllotoxin and vinblastine are known to depolymerize microtubules in cells.

Colchicine inhibits microtubule polymerization by binding to tubulin. It can therefore act as a spindle poison (tubulin is required for mitosis) and can act in mitosis. In view of this, it can act on cancer cells but its value is limited in chemotherapy due to its toxicity against normal cells.

6a. False – it is aspiration of fetal chorionic villi and not amniotic fluid.
6b. False – it can be done by either the abdominal or the vaginal route.
6c. True – CVS is performed after 9 weeks.
6d. True
6e. True – placental mosaicism creates confusion in the diagnosis.

7a. True
7b. False – HbF – $\alpha_2\gamma_2$
7c. True
7d. False – HbA_2 – $\alpha_2\delta_2$
7e. True

Note
There are six globin polypeptide chains in humans – α, β, γ, δ, ϵ and ζ. Each chain has a specific amino acid chain linked by peptide bonds. The α chain has

141 amino acids and the β, γ and δ chains each have 146 amino acids. The last two (ϵ, ζ) are found in embryonic erythrocytes.

Approximately ninety-eight per cent of the total haemoglobin in normal adults is HbA ($\alpha_2\beta_2$) and HbA_2 is around 2.5%.

HbF ($\alpha_2\gamma_2$) is the haemoglobin in newborns (50–85%) and declines rapidly to 10–15% at 4 months of age. Gower 1, Gower 2 and Portland haemoglobin are found before 7–10 weeks of gestational age and are embryonic haemoglobin.

HbH Barts is a tetramer of β and γ chains, respectively, and has poor function in O_2 transport. Some abnormality in the haemoglobin molecule would lead to haemoglobinopathies, e.g. sickle cell disease (HbS). Under low O_2 tension, the red cells acquire an abnormal shape. In the sixth amino acid from the N-terminal in the β chain, valine replaces the glutamic acid of the normal haemoglobin (HbA).

8a. True
8b. False – it is associated with micrognathia.
8c. False
8d. True
8e. False

Note
The other features of trisomy 18 or Edwards syndrome include deformed ears, overlapping fingers, growth retardation and premature death.

The features of trisomy 21 include hypotonia, small ears, upward and outward slanting of the palpebral fissures, Brushfield spots on the iris and a flat nape of the neck.

9a. True
9b. True
9c. True
9d. False
9e. False

Note
- Trisomy 21 – Down syndrome.
- Trisomy 18 – Edwards syndrome.
- Trisomy 13 – Patau syndrome.
- Cri–du–chat syndrome is due to deletion of a portion of the short arm of chromosome 5 (characteristic features seen in children are learning disability, microcephaly, typical facial features and hypertelorism).

10a. True
10b. False – it does not play a major role in tissue transplantation.
10c. False
10d. True
10e. True

11a. True
11b. False – is an X-linked condition.
11c. False – is an X-linked condition.
11d. False – is an X-linked condition.
11e. True

12a. True
12b. False
12c. True
12d. False
12e. False

Note
During conception mitochondrial DNA is transmitted to the offspring via the ovum, so the trait is transmitted from females to all her children and from males to none of his children. Spermatozoa do not contribute mitochondria to the zygote.

13a. False – is an autosomal recessive condition.
13b. True – pleiotropy is a phenomenon where a single gene is responsible for several affects.
13c. True
13d. False – there is a deficiency of phenylalanine hydroxylase.
13e. False – the conversion of phenylalanine to tyrosine is lacking and therefore there is an accumulation of phenylalanine in the blood (detected by the Guthrie test). There is increased excretion of phenylpyruvic acid in the urine (ferric chloride test). The treatment is a phenylalanine-free diet.

Note
The manifestations of phenylketonuria in an untreated child include severe learning disability, microcephaly, decreased melanin production, blonde hair and blue eyes. The enzyme phenylalanine hydroxylase cannot be replaced, thus removal of phenylalanine from diet is the main modality of treatment.

14a. True
14b. True
14c. True
14d. False – sickle cell disease is a type of inherited blood disorder that affects the red blood cells (RBCs). These RBCs tend to sickle (contain abnormal haemoglobin 'S') when exposed to low oxygen tension or hypoxia and consequently are not mouldable like the normal RBCs, thus blocking the small capillaries (leading to sickle cell crises). The mutation in the haemoglobin gene causes this condition (homozygosity in the mutation causes sickle cell disease (HbSS) and heterozygosity in the mutation causes sickle cell trait – HbAS).
14e. True

15a. True
15b. True
15c. False
15d. True
15e. True

Note
Examples of X-linked recessive inheritance include haemophilia, glucose 6-phosphate dehydrogenase deficiency (G6PD), Duchenne muscular dystrophy and partial colour blindness (not able to distinguish between red and green shades).

16a. True
16b. False – mitochondria contain enzymes for the citric acid cycle.
16c. True
16d. True
16e. True

Note
Peroxisome is a membrane-bound organelle and contains different enzymes. It is formed in the rough endoplasmic reticulum and matures in the Golgi apparatus. It contains enzymes for β-oxidation of fatty acids. It also produces hydrogen peroxide (H_2O_2) for the destruction of microorganisms phagocytosed by the cell. The catalase contained in it converts toxic H_2O_2 to non-toxic water and oxygen.

17a. False – prevalence is 7:1000.
17b. True
17c. True
17d. True
17e. True

Note
When one member of an allelic pair is able to express, it is called autosomal dominant inheritance. Therefore it can be expressed in the heterozygous as well as the homozygous state. It can have variable expressions with minor-to-severe abnormalities. The trait appears in every generation. Fifty per cent of the children would be affected irrespective of the sex of the child.

18a. False – its inheritance is autosomal recessive.
18b. True
18c. True
18d. False – its inheritance is autosomal recessive.
18e. True

Note
The other examples of autosomal dominant diseases include:

- osteogenesis imperfecta.
- Huntington's disease.
- neurofibromatosis type 1.
- haemochromatosis.
- baldness in males.

19a. False – the transmission of the trait is not influenced by the sex.
19b. False – unaffected individual does not transmit the trait to their children.
19c. True
19d. True
19e. False – males and females have an equal chance of getting the trait as well as transmitting it.

20a. True
20b. True
20c. False – it is a rare genetic disease (the majority are caused by deletion on chromosome 15 which is inherited from the father and the rest are caused by inheriting two chromosome 15 from the mother) first described by Swiss doctors A. Prader, A. Labhart and H. Willi. It is characterized by obesity (due to over-eating and increased appetite), excessive eating (hyperphagia), short stature, small hands and feet, hypotonia and hypogonadism.
20d. False – Meigs syndrome is a triad of benign ovarian fibroma or tumour, ascites and right-sided pleural effusion. Resolution occurs once the tumour has been removed.
20e. True

21a. True
21b. True
21c. False – a carrier is phenotypically normal.
21d. False – it usually involves chromosome 14. Most of the interchanges are between chromosomes 13 and 14.
21e. True

22a. False – prevalence is 2.5:1000.
22b. False – it is expressed in the homozygous state.
22c. True
22d. True
22e. True

Note
Examples of autosomal recessive conditions include:

- albinism
- cystic fibrosis
- congenital adrenal hyperplasia
- galactosaemia
- Gaucher disease
- haemoglobinopathies
- mucopolysaccharidoses (e.g. Hurler syndrome type I)
- Niemann–Pick disease
- pentosuria
- phenylketonuria
- Tay–Sachs disease
- Wilson disease.

23a. True
23b. True
23c. False
23d. True
23e. True

Note
The other conditions with granuloma formation are leprosy, TB, sarcoidosis, etc. There is chronic inflammation in these conditions and macrophages are the main type of cell type seen in such areas.

24a. True
24b. True
24c. False – is an X-linked dominant condition.
24d. False – is an autosomal recessive condition.
24e. True

25a. False – is an X-linked recessive condition.
25b. True
25c. True
25d. False – is a Y-linked condition.
25e. False – is an X-linked recessive condition.

26a. True
26b. True
26c. False – it is vice versa.
26d. False – all the daughters will be affected. (If an affected male marries a normal female, all the daughters will be affected but none of the sons will be affected.)
26e. True

27a. False – they are formed in rough endoplasmic reticulum.
27b. True
17c. False – primary lysosomes emerge from the Golgi apparatus.
27d. False – they do not take part in metabolic events.
27e. True

28a. True
28b. False
28c. True
28d. False
28e. False

Note
Staphylococcus aureus is the most common organism causing toxic shock syndrome and is mainly seen in women who used tampons during menstrual periods. They usually present with high temperature, hypotension and desquamating rash involving the palms and soles. In addition to the above organs it involves other organs in the body.

29a. True
29b. True
29c. True
29d. True
29e. True

Note
The other cells that can regenerate include myofibres, lining of the uterus, cells of the seminiferous tubules and most neurons in the body.

30a. True
30b. True
30c. False
30d. True
30e. True

Note
The following are chemical carcinogens other than the ones mentioned above: soots, tars (skin cancer), cigarette smoking (lung cancer), benzidine (bladder cancer), arsenic (skin cancer), nickel (lung cancer) and vinyl chloride (liver cancer).

31a. True
31b. False – it is a slow growing tumour.
31c. False
31d. True
31e. True

Note
Carcinoid tumour is a malignant tumour that secretes 5HT. 5HT is destroyed in liver. It can cause diarrhoea, flushing, bronchospasm and facial telangiectasia. It can occur in ovarian teratoma with carcinoid component.

32a. True – vWf is a blood glycoprotein involved in haemostasis. Its deficiency causes Von Willebrand disease.
32b. True
32c. True
32d. False – increases the half-life of factor VIII.
32e. False

33a. True – decrease in pH shifts the curve to the right.
33b. False – shifts to the right occur in conditions with high $PaCO_2$ levels.
33c. False
33d. True
33e. True

Note
Unloading more O_2 at the tissues due to decreased affinity of O_2 for haemoglobin is called the Bohr effect (seen when there is a shift to the right with the haemoglobin dissociation curve).

34a. False – the primary immune response produces IgM.
34b. False
34c. True
34d. False – the secretory immunogobulin is IgA. It is seen in mucosal secretions such as saliva and genitourinary and bronchial secretions. It is also seen in colostrum.
34e. False – IgG crosses the placenta.

35a. True – C3 is a major opsonin and its deficiency results in recurrent pyogenic infections, especially with capsulate bacteria.
35b. False – C1, C2 and C4 deficiencies are associated with autoimmune diseases such as SLE and do not usually predispose individuals to severe infections.
35c. True
35d. True – C1 esterase deficiency causes overactivation of the complement system with resultant damaging inflammatory effects. This is thought to be the causative factor in the development of angioneurotic oedema and paroxysmal nocturnal haemoglobinuria.
35e. True

Note
A group of serum proteins that work with antibody activity to destroy pathogens is called a complement. It is produced by hepatocytes and macrophages and is part of the innate immunity. It stimulates inflammation and promotes phagocytosis of antigens when exposed to a pathogen. Some complements act as proenzymes which when activated become proteases to start off a cascade of reactions (the classic complement cascade is activated by antigen-bound IgG and IgM while the alternative complement cascade is activated by molecules on the bacterial cell surface). Thus its deficiency causes certain disorders or diseases depending on the type of complement deficiency.

36a. True
36b. False – type II collagen is seen in cartilage and type I collagen is seen in skin, bones and tendons.
36c. True
36d. False – type IV collagen is exclusively seen in the basement membrane.
36e. True

37a. False – tortuous glands are seen in the secretory phase.
37b. False – simple tubular glands are seen in the proliferative phase.
37c. True
37d. False – stroma is highly cellular in the secretory phase.
37e. True

Note
Various changes occur in the endometrium during the menstrual cycle. It is divided into proliferative and secretory phases. During the proliferative phase, under the influence of oestrogen, the endometrium thickens and invaginates to form simple tubular glands. The blood supply to the

endometrium is derived from the spiral artery. These glands subsequently become tortuous and glycogen rich during the secretory phase under the influence of progesterone. The stroma becomes highly vascular and the endometrium is ready to accept if conception occurs. Without conception and implantation, the corpus luteum degenerates and the stratum functionalis layer is shed as the menstrual period. The basal layer of the endometrium helps in regeneration of the endometrium.

38a. True – coeliac disease is also called gluten-sensitive enteropathy. It is due to an autoimmune inflammatory reaction of the small intestine to a wheat protein called gluten in someone who is genetically susceptible. The treatment is gluten-free diet.
38b. True
38c. True
38d. True
38e. True

Note
The inability of the lining of the gut to absorb nutrients into the bloodstream is called malabsorption. Other causes of malabsorption include lactose intolerance (inability to digest sugar lactose in milk), acrodermatitis enteropathica and biliary atresia.

39a. True – erythema nodosum is seen in ulcerative colitis and sarcoidosis.
39b. False – erythema chronicum migrans is seen in Lyme disease (caused by organism *Borrelia burgdoferi*).
39c. True
39d. False
39e. False – hyperpigmentation is seen in Addison disease.

40a. False – more common in young adults.
40b. True
40c. True
40d. True
40e. False – it is more often seen in women.

41a. True
41b. True
41c. False – the distinctive feature of apoptosis is synthesis of RNA and proteins prior to cell death.
41d. True
41e. False – it involves both single and multiple cells.

42a. True – muscle also stores glycogen.
42b. True
42c. True
42d. False – during exercise the glycogen in the muscle supplies energy for muscle contraction.
42e. True

43a. False
43b. True
43c. True
43d. False
43e. True

Note
Type I collagen – skin (mature collagen in dermis), sclera, cornea, blood vessels, tendon, ligament, bone and hollow organs. Disorder of type I collagen leads to osteogenesis imperfecta and Ehlers–Danlos syndrome.
Type 2 collagen – cartilage and notochord of embryos.
Type 3 – strengthens the walls of hollow structures (arteries, intestines and uterus). Also found in early scar tissue. Disorder of type 3 collagen leads to Ehlers–Danlos syndrome.
Type 4 collagen – basement membrane and lens of the eye. Disorder of type 4 collagen leads to Alport syndrome.
Type 5 collagen – fetal tissue, placenta and interstitial tissue.
Type 7 collagen – present in the junctions between epithelium and mesenchyma (anchoring tissues).

44a. True
44b. False – it inhibits glucagon release.
44c. True
44d. False – growth hormone is stimulated by amino acids, hypoglycaemia and stress.
44e. True

45a. True
45b. True
45c. True
45d. False – carbohydrates and fatty acids are the normal energy sources.
45e. True

Note
ATP is required for both transport and maintenance of ionic gradients.

46a. True – monosaccharides, fatty acids and amino acids are metabolized to produce acetate in the form of acetyl-CoA.
46b. True
46c. False – it enters the citric acid cycle.
46d. True
46e. False – it is converted to 6 molecules of CO_2 and 24 atoms of hydrogen.

47a. False
47b. True
47c. True
47d. False – one molecule of glucose is converted to two molecules of pyruvic acid.
47e. True – ATP is converted to ADP; thus it is energy dependent.

48a. True
48b. False – this step is not energy dependent. Glucose 6-phosphate is isomerized to fructose 6-phosphate.
48c. False – it produces energy (ATP).
48d. False – it produces energy (ATP).
48e. True

Note
In the glycolytic pathway two ATP molecules are used in the first half of the cycle and four are formed in the second half of the cycle, with an overall gain of two ATP molecules.

49a. True
49b. False – it is inhibited by citrate.
49c. False – it is inhibited by high concentrations of ATP.
49d. False
49e. True

Note
It is a rate-limiting step in the glycolytic pathway.

50a. True
50b. False
50c. True – the nucleus of a hydrogen atom is part of the NAD (nicotinamide adenine dinucleotide) molecule.
50d. True
50e. True

51a. False – it contains high intrinsic energy.
51b. True – when it is fed into the electron transport chain, it needs oxygen to provide energy (in the form of ATP).
51c. True
51d. True
51e. True

52a. True
52b. False – is the end-product of aerobic glycolysis and is derived from phosphoenolpyruvate.
52c. True
52d. True
52e. True

53a. False – it is allosterically activated by fructose 1,6-diphosphate.
53b. False – the enzyme pyruvate kinase is involved in glycolysis. It catalyses the transfer of phosphate from phosphoenolpyruvate to adenosine diphosphate (ADP), producing one molecule of adenosine triphosphate (ATP) and pyruvate.
53c. True
53d. True
53e. False – it is inhibited by glucagon in the fasting state where pyruvate kinase is phosphorylated, and therefore the conversion of phosphoenolpyruvate to pyruvate is prevented. Instead it is converted to glucose and provides glucose to various organs in the fasting state.

Note
The conversion of phosphoenolpyruvate to pyruvate is the final step in the glycolytic pathway. This action is catalysed by pyruvate kinase.

54a. False
54b. False – it is restricted to erythrocytes.
54c. True
54d. True
54e. True

Note
It is the second most common cause of enzyme deficiency-related haemolytic anaemia after glucose-6-phosphate dehydrogenase deficiency. It accounts for 95% of all inherited defects in glycolytic enzymes. It can cause both mild and severe haemolytic anaemia.

55a. False – it is composed of four globin chains (two alpha and two beta) and one haem ring.
55b. False – the haem ring is synthesized in mitochondria.
55c. False
55d. False – supply of iron could be a rate-limiting step in haem synthesis.
55e. True

56a. True
56b. True
56c. False – the deficiency is an X-linked dominant condition.
56d. True
56e. True

Note
Pyruvate dehydrogenase complex oxidatively decarboxylates pyruvate to acetyl-CoA. Its deficiency is the most common cause of biochemical congenital lactic acidosis. Arsenic poisoning inactivates the enzyme by binding to lipoic acid.

57a. True
57b. False
57c. False
57d. True
57e. True

Note
The electron transport system or the respiratory chain is located in the mitochondria. As the inner mitochondrial membrane is impermeable to reduced nicotinamide adenine dinucleotide (NADH), the cell uses a biochemical system (malate–aspartate shuttle) to transfer electrons across to the inner membrane of the mitochondria. This allows the transfer of electrons from NADH in the cytoplasm to NAD^+ in the matrix to generate ATP (one molecule of NADH has the potential to generate three molecules of ATP from ADP).

58a. False
58b. False
58c. False
58d. True
58e. True

Note
The cAMP (adenosine cyclic monophosphate) is synthesized from ATP (adenosine triphosphate). It is rapidly and continually degraded by cAMP phosphodiesterases. It activates the enzyme protein kinase A. The activity of adenylyl cyclase is regulated by the trimeric G-protein. The transfer of the terminal phosphate group from ATP to specific serine or threonine molecules of particular proteins is catalysed by protein kinase A.

59a. False
59b. False
59c. False
59d. True
59e. True

Note
Potassium is mainly intracellular. Around 98% of total body potassium is intracellular. Only 2% is extracellular. Acidosis, hypertonicity and cell death would lead to potassium loss from a cell. Alkalosis and insulin promote potassium influx into the cell.

60a. True – the brain uses more ketones, β-hydroxybutyrate and acetoacetate to produce oxidative energy during fasting.
60b. True
60c. True
60d. False
60e. True

61a. True
61b. True
61c. True
61d. False – cyclooxygenase converts PGG_2 to PGH_2.
61e. True

Note
The basic derivative for prostaglandin synthesis is arachidonic acid. Arachidonic acid is released from membrane phospholipids (glycerophospholipids), the release of which is promoted by phospholipase A_2, phospholipase C and diacylglycerol lipases. Cyclooxygenase also promotes conversion of arachidonic acid to PGG_2. Prostaglandin isomerases convert PGH_2 to $PGF_{2\alpha}$ and PGE_2.

62a. False – it is produced by L-arginine.
62b. False – it has a short half-life of 5–10 seconds.
62c. True
62d. False – during pregnancy increased nitric oxide is thought to mediate vasodilatation and also promotes a fall in blood pressure.
62e. True

Note
Nitric oxide synthase promotes the formation of nitric oxide from L-arginine. The enzyme requires cofactors and oxygen to facilitate this action. It is converted to nitrates and nitrites in the blood. In the smooth muscle, it promotes production of cGMP (guanosine cyclic monophosphate) by binding to iron in the active site of the enzyme guanylyl cyclase (which induces smooth muscle relaxation).

63a. False
63b. True
63c. True
63d. True
63e. False – in humans, most amino acid detoxification occurs in the liver.

64a. True
64b. False
64c. True
64d. True
64e. False – dopamine is hydroxylated to noradrenaline.

Note
Pathway: phenylalanine → tyrosine → dopa → dopamine → noradrenaline → adrenaline.

65a. False – they contain less oxygen than carbohydrates.
65b. True
65c. True
65d. False – they yield more than twice the energy on oxidation than from an equivalent amount of carbohydrates.
65e. True

66a. False
66b. True
66c. False
66d. True
66e. False

Note
Cervical intraepithelial neoplasia (CIN) is a histological diagnosis characterized by large abnormal nuclei and reduced cell cytoplasm. There is loss of the cellular stratification and maturation throughout the thickness of the cervical epithelium with increased mitotic activity. The extent of the above features identifies the degree of CIN. If the mitoses and immature cells are present only in the lower one-third of the epithelium, the lesion is designed at CIN I (low-grade lesion), whereas involvement of the middle and upper thirds is classed as CIN II and CIN III (high-grade lesion), respectively.

Women with cervical dyskaryosis are usually asymptomatic but those with invasive disease can present with an offensive vaginal discharge, intermenstrual bleeding, postcoital or postmenopausal bleeding. So these symptoms warrant further investigation to rule out any cervical pathology. The degree of dyskaryosis (mild to severe) often correlates with the changes that are found at histology (CIN I, CIN II and CIN III). However, this may not always be the case (mild dyskaryosis may be associated with a high-grade lesion on colposcopy).

The majority of the abnormalities are minor abnormalities on cytology for cervical screening (borderline and mild dyskaryosis) in the UK. The treatment depends on the grade of the lesion (low grade or high grade) on colposcopy and confirmation of the same on biopsy (histology). CIN I may regress spontaneously in many cases and so does not necessarily require treatment but definitely needs follow-up with cytological screening. Obviously, if the abnormality persists or progresses to a higher degree, treatment needs to be undertaken.

67a. False
67b. False
67c. True
67d. True
67e. True

Note
The squamocolumnar junction is located within the endocervical canal before puberty, but as a result of the hormonal changes at puberty there is eversion of the columnar epithelium towards the vagina. Simultaneously, there is change in the vaginal pH (becomes more acidic, pH 4–5). This results in 'metaplasia' whereby the everted columnar epithelium changes to squamous epithelium. This area is called the transformation zone (TZ). Most precancerous changes occur in this area and therefore it is important that the squamocolumnar junction is sampled when taking a smear.

68a. True
68b. False
68c. True
68d. False – is conversion of columnar to squamous epithelium.
68e. False

Note
Metaplasia is a physiological process. It is not caused by either herpes simplex virus or human papillomavirus. It is promoted by changes in the vaginal pH (becomes more acidic) at puberty.

69a. False
69b. True
69c. True
69d. True
69e. True

Note
According to NHS Cervical Screening Programme guidelines, the following are the criteria for referral to a colposcopy clinic.

1. Three inadequate samples.
   The smear is inadequate for interpretation in the laboratory to give any definitive diagnosis. This could be due to a poorly prepared smear or it may not contain the right type of cells (not representative of transformation zone). The rate of inadequate smears is reduced with the introduction of liquid-based cytology (LBC).
2. Three smear tests reported as borderline nuclear changes in squamous cells.
   The smear is interpreted as borderline either when it is difficult to differentiate between HPV changes or mild dyskaryosis or where it is difficult to differentiate benign or reactive changes from significant degrees of dyskaryosis.
3. One smear test reported as borderline nuclear change in endocervical cells. This indicates borderline glandular changes in endocervical cells. Glandular changes in the endocervical cells are often associated with cervical intraepithelial neoplasia and an underlying malignancy (adenocarcinoma) must not be overlooked.
4. One smear report of mild dyskaryosis.
5. One smear report of moderate or severe dyskaryosis.
6. One smear test reported as possible invasion.
7. One test reported as glandular neoplasia.
8. Suspicious-looking cervix.

Reference:
Luesley D, Leeson S (eds). *Colposcopy and Pragramme Management: Guidelines for the NHS Cervical Screening Programme*, NHSCSP Publication No. 20. Sheffield: NHS Cancer Screening Programmes, 2004. Available at: www.bsccp.org.uk/docs/public/pdf/nhscsp20.pdf.

70a. True
70b. True
70c. True
70d. True
70e. True

Note

Acetowhite epithelium is the appearance described after the application of acetic acid during colposcopic examination. It is caused by precipitation of nuclear proteins (due to increased nuclear density) and is a transient phenomenon. It can be seen in various conditions quoted in question 70. The intensity of whiteness increases with the degree of CIN, e.g. CIN1 (mild acetowhite area) to CIN3 (dense acetowhite area). The other features of CIN on colposcopy are mosaicism and punctation. The satellite lesions away from the transformation zone (TZ) on the cervix usually indicate HPV infection.

71a. True
71b. False
71c. True
71d. True
71e. True

Note

FISH is used for the detection of submicroscopic chromosomal deletions and is also used to assist with the identification of subtle translocations and chromosome markers. It can be performed on metaphase preparations from cultured amniocytes and chorionic villi and also on interphase nuclei from amniotic fluid and blood. The latter is used in prenatal diagnosis when a fetal abnormality is detected, e.g. aneuploidies such as trisomy 21.

72a. True – is associated with short stature, characteristic facies, hypotonia, obesity and learning disability.
72b. False
72c. True – is associated with an ataxic gait, seizures and learning disability.
72d. True – is associated with cleft palate, cardiac defects, hypocalcaemia and learning difficulties.
72e. False

Note

Microdeletion syndromes are disorders that arise due to submicroscopic deletions of the chromosomes. These can be detected by fluorescence *in situ* hybridization techniques. The other syndromes due to microdeletion include Miller–Dieker (associated with lissencephaly, characteristic facies) and Williams syndrome (associated with hypocalcaemia, learning disability, characteristic facies and supravalvular aortic stenosis).

73a. False
73b. True
73c. True
73d. False
73e. False

Note
There are two types of immunity. (1) Innate or non-specific immunity – this includes the innate (inbuilt) immune system, e.g. skin acts as a mechanical, physical, anatomical barrier against most organisms. This is not antigen specific or antigen dependent. (2) Specific immunity – this is in response to a specific antigen and the response is antigen dependent. There is a definite lag period between the antigen exposure and time of maximal response.

74a. False – they resemble lymphocytes in their morphology.
74b. True
74c. False – CD3 cell surface marker is absent.
74d. True
74e. True

Note
Natural killer cells play a role in innate immunity along with other cells (e.g. activated macrophages). They become lymphokine-activated cells on exposure to interleukin 2 (IL-2) and interferon-γ, which are capable of killing malignant cells. This is the basis of using these cells in cancer therapy.

75a. False – they are serum proteins acting as antibodies (an important defence mechanism against microorganisms) and are produced by plasma cells.
75b. True – polypeptide chains are made of two identical light chains and two identical heavy chains. These are held together by disulphide bonds.
75c. False – the light chains are kappa (κ) and lambda (λ). The light chains are alike in all classes of immunoglobulins.
75d. False – the heavy chains differ in each immunoglobulin.
75e. True – immunoglobulins have a special structure and are made of a variable (concerned with antigen binding) and a constant region (concerned with complement fixation).

76a. False
76b. False
76c. True
76d. True
76e. True

Note
Necrosis is death of a cell or group of cells or a part of a tissue or whole organ in a particular part of the body. This can be due to some sort of insult, e.g. ischaemia, bacterial infections and toxins, physical or chemical agents, and radiation.

Examples
Caseation necrosis – is mainly described in the context of tuberculosis.

Aseptic necrosis – is described in relation to the head of femur after traumatic hip dislocation. In this condition necrosis occurs without infection.

Coagulative necrosis is seen in hypoxic conditions leading to infarction. Myocardial infarction also indicates tissue necrosis where death or necrosis of the heart muscle occurs due to lack of oxygen supply in the affected part. The exception is brain where ischaemia causes liquefaction necrosis.

Liquefactive necrosis is associated with destruction of the cells and pus formation and is typically seen in bacterial infections due to extensive inflammatory reaction.

Fatty necrosis is the death of fatty tissue by the action of the enzyme lipase, e.g. acute pancreatitis.

77a. True
77b. True – it acts only after the formation of an antigen–antibody complex and as a result causes lysis of the antigen-bearing cell by a series of reactions.
77c. True
77d. False – is associated with production of inflammation and rejection of the implanted tissue or organ.
77e. True

78a. True
78b. False – the greater the antigen similarity, the less the chance of graft rejection and vice versa.
78c. True – the following changes occur in a recipient in response to the grafted tissue. First there is cellular proliferation in the regional lymph nodes of the host. The cells that are formed are small lymphocytes (T cells and B cells). T cells (thymus-dependent cells) promote tissue rejection by cell-mediated reactions. T cells respond by proliferation and differentiation to form lymphoblasts. These blast cells gives rise to T-effector cells, T-suppressor cells and T-helper cells. T-effector cells react with the graft site and lead to rejection.
78d. False – homograft rejection does not occur in identical twins.
78e. False – it does not occur in non-identical twins where mixing of the placental circulation has taken place *in utero.*

79a. True – e.g. skin graft from thigh to face in the same individual.
79b. False – this is a tissue graft from a donor to a host with the same genotype, e.g. tissue graft between identical twins.
79c. False – this is a tissue graft from a donor to a host with a different genotype but a member of the same species.
79d. True – an example is a graft between animals and humans.
79e. True

80a. False – is divided into three classes (class I, II and III).
80b. True
80c. True – class I molecules present the foreign antigens on the surface of infected cells and thus are responsible for transplant rejection.
80d. False – class II molecules are present on the surface of B cells and phagocytes (antigen-presenting cells of the immune system).
80e. False – class III region codes for the complement protein.

Note
MHC region is divided into three subgroups:

– MHC class I
– MHC class II
– MHC class III.

They display both self- and non-self antigens on the cell surface (the proteins encoded by the MHC are expressed on the surface of the cells).

81a. True
81b. True
81c. True
81d. False
81e. True

Note
The class I and class II molecules are expressed on cells and tissues whereas class III molecules are represented on proteins in serum and other body fluids. MHC is composed of human leucocyte antigen (HLA) genes. Class I molecules are expressed on all nucleated cells and platelets.

82a. True
82b. False
82c. True
82d. False
82e. True

Note
BCG does not prevent pulmonary tuberculosis but reduces dissemination. Hepatitis B vaccine contains only surface proteins of the virus.

83a. True
83b. False
83c. False
83d. False
83e. False

Note
Live attenuated vaccines generally should be avoided in immunocompromised people, and these would include measles, mumps, rubella, polio (Sabin), varicella, yellow fever, BCG and oral typhoid. Killed vaccines and subunit vaccines can be administered.

84a. True – direct Coombs test is positive as maternal antibodies are already bound to fetal red blood cells.
84b. True
84c. True
84d. False – as bilurubin is excreted through the placenta during intrauterine life, jaundice does not appear immediately at birth. The fetal RBCs are destroyed in the reticuloendothelial system (RES) as maternal antibodies are bound to fetal RBCs. This causes an increase in the bilurubin in neonatal blood resulting in jaundice (develops after 24 hours).
84e. False – it is characterized by the presence of erythroblasts in the cord blood.

85a. True
85b. True – also lead to development of a female.
85c. False – the absence of Y chromosome leads to development of a female.
85d. True
85e. False – The presence of Y chromosome leads to development of a male irrespective of the number of X chromosomes, e.g. 48XXXY.

86a. False – DHT is derived from testosterone.
86b. False – 5α-reductase is required for the formation of dihydrotestosterone from testosterone.
86c. True – this happens around 12–14 weeks of pregnancy. It causes the genital tubercle to enlarge to form the penis and genital swellings fuse to form the scrotum.
86d. True – the deficiency leads to formation of female external genitalia and male internal genitalia (testis is present).
86e. True

87a. True – 46 paternal chromosomes (derived either from dispermy or due to duplication of the haploid sperm chromosome) and 23 maternal chromosomes.
87b. False – maternal and paternal origin.
87c. False – fertilization of an ovum by two sperm results in partial mole.
87d. False – fertilization of an empty ovum by two sperm results in a complete mole.
87e. True

88a. False – Sex chromatin is derived from one of the X chromosomes and is attached to the nuclear membrane. It is used for sex determination (seen as a Barr body in the cells of the epidermis, oral mucosa, amniotic fluid and drumstick in the leucocytes). The number of Barr bodies at interphase is equal to number of X chromosomes minus one (nX – 1).
Sex chromatin appears in the extra-embryonic membranes at about day 12 and by about day 16 in the embryo. It is absent in female germ cells and oocytes.
88b. False – stains heavily (darkly) with basic dyes.

88c. False – it is seen at the interphase.
88d. True
88e. True

89a. True – the other X chromosome is inactivated and small. Sex chromatin is present in females and absent in males.
89b. False – it occurs in embryonic life.
89c. False
89d. False – in different cells of the same individual, inactivation of the X chromosome is random and can be of either maternal or paternal origin.
89e. True

90a. False – this occurs during the metaphase.
90b. True
90c. True
90d. False – this occurs during the prophase.
90e. False – this occurs during the telophase.

Note
Mitosis occurs in the somatic cells and is divided into four phases – prophase, metaphase, anaphase and telophase.

91a. True – any penetatrating ionizing radiation induces mutational change, e.g. X-rays, radioactive substances, neutrons from nuclear reaction.
91b. True
91c. True
91d. True
91e. True

Note
Mutations may also occur spontaneously without any inducing mutagenic agent. Mutagenic agents have a direct effect in the cells on which they act.

92a. True
92b. True
92c. True
92d. True
92e. False – sickle cell disease does not offer protection against malaria. People with sickle cell disease are susceptible to death due to complications of this disease.

Note
HLA-B53 and interleukin-4 are associated with a low risk of severe malaria.

The following red cell defences against malaria are:
Haemoglobin C
Haemoglobin S
β-thalassaemia
Glucose 6-phosphate dehydrogenase deficiency.

93a. True
93b. False
93c. False
93d. False
93e. True

Note
Lead I is the signal between the aVR electrode (on the right arm) and the aVL electrode (on the left arm). Lead II is between the aVR electrode (on the right arm) and the aVF electrode (on the left leg). Lead III is between the aVL electrode (on the left arm) and the aVF electrode (on the left leg). Lead aVR has the positive electrode on the right arm. The negative electrode is a combination of the left arm electrode and the left leg (red) electrode, which 'augments' the signal strength of the positive electrode on the right arm. Leads aVL and aVF are corresponding combinations with the left arm and left foot and combinations of other leads. Lead V1 is placed in the fourth intercostal space (between ribs 4 and 5) to the right of the sternum (breastbone) and V2 in the fourth intercostal space (between ribs 4 and 5) to the left of the sternum. The P–R interval is measured from the beginning of the P wave to the beginning of the QRS complex. It is usually 120–200 milliseconds. Left axis deviation is considered normal in pregnant women.

94a. False
94b. True
94c. False
94d. True
94e. True

Note
The most commonly used abdominal probe operates at a frequency of 3.5 MHz whereas the transvaginal probe operates at between 6 and 7.5 MHz.

The choice of frequency is a trade-off between axial resolution of the image and imaging depth: lower frequencies (longer wavelength) produce less resolution but image deeper into the body. Lateral resolution is mediated by the beam width.

95a. False
95b. False
95c. True
95d. False
95e. True

Note
Continuous-wave Doppler ultrasound transmits and receives ultrasound continuously and is not range specific, so it is difficult to isolate the Doppler signals from a particular vessel. Pulsed-wave (PW) Doppler ultrasound transmits short pulses of ultrasound, the echoes of which are received after a short interval of time, and thus allows measurement of the depth at which blood flow is observed. Also, the size of the sample volume can be changed. Pulsed-wave Doppler ultrasound is more commonly used in

obstetrics and gynaecology due to these advantages. Continuous-wave Doppler ultrasound is used in adult cardiology to investigate high velocities in the aorta.

Colour Doppler imaging produces a colour-coded map of Doppler frequency shifts superimposed on a B-mode ultrasound image. Red colour stands for Doppler shifts towards the transducer and blue for shifts away from it.

Ambiguity of the Doppler shift is known as aliasing and affects the pulsed-wave Doppler system. When pulses are transmitted at a given sampling frequency called the pulse repetition frequency (PRF), the maximum Doppler frequency shift that can be measured unambiguously is half the PRF. If the blood velocity and the flow angle being measured combine to give a frequency shift greater than half the PRF, then aliasing occurs.

Doppler frequency is affected by three factors: blood flow velocity, ultrasound frequency and the angle of insonation.

When an ultrasound pulse travels through the tissues, there is a temperature rise as some of the pulses absorbed by the tissues are converted to heat. The thermal index (TI) and mechanical index (MI) are indices used to protect the patients from excessive exposure. TIS (soft-tissue thermal index) is monitored during scans carried out during the first 8 weeks after conception and TIB (bone thermal index) thereafter. Thermal effects are due to heating of the tissues, and mechanical effects are due to cavitation and streaming in fluids plus stress at tissue interfaces. A TI <0.5 and MI <0.3 are advocated by the Safety Group of the British Medical Ultrasound Society.

96a. True
96b. True – intra-abdominal pressure minus intravesical pressure gives detrusor pressure.
96c. True
96d. True
96e. False

Note
Free uroflowmetry measures how fast the patient can empty his or her bladder. Multichannel cystometry measures the pressure in the rectum and in the bladder, using two pressure catheters, to deduce the vesical pressure and the presence of contractions of the bladder wall, during bladder filling or other provocative manouevres. The strength of the urethra can also be tested during this phase, using a cough or Valsalva manoeuvre, to confirm genuine stress incontinence. Pressure uroflowmetry also measures the rate of voiding, but with simultaneous assessment of bladder and rectal pressures. It helps demonstrate the reasons for difficulty in voiding, for example bladder muscle weakness or obstruction of the bladder outflow.

97a. False
97b. True
97c. True

97d. False
97e. True

Note
In bipolar diathermy the current flows between the electrodes and does not run through the body. Therefore a return electrode is not required.

With unipolar diathermy the current runs from the electrode, preferentially through the vascular tree towards the return electrode (usually located over the quadriceps muscle). If there is poor contact, burns will occur on the skin at the site of the return electrode. Burns are therefore more common.

To minimize the effects of muscle and neural stimulation, electrosurgical equipment typically operates at a frequency of 100 kHz to 5 MHz.

98a. True
98b. False
98c. True
98d. True
98e. False

Note
Forms of ionizing radiation:

Alpha particles (rays)	Helium nuclei (two protons, two neutrons)
Beta particles (rays)	Electrons
Gamma rays	Photons (electromagnetic radiation)
X-rays	Photons (electromagnetic radiation)
Protons	Positive charge
Neutrons	Neutral charge

Particles release high doses of radiation but have very low penetration whereas electromagnetic radiation has less radiation but more penetration. Radiation relies on ionization of local oxygen; it therefore works better in well-oxygenated tumours with less necrosis. Oxygen free radicals cause more damage to exposed DNA and therefore work better in rapidly dividing tissues.

99a. False
99b. True
99c. False
99d. True
99e. False

Note
Computed tomography (CT) scans subject the client to a dose of radiation 50–60 times that of a chest radiograph. In 2000–2001, CT scans constituted 7% of all radiology examinations, but contributed 47% of the total collective dose from medical X-ray examinations. Ventilation–perfusion ($\dot{V}/\dot{Q}$) scans increase the risk of developing childhood cancer for the fetus. CT pulmonary angiogram (CTPA) increases the risk of breast cancer in the mother by an estimated 13.6%.

No adverse effects of MRI on the fetus have been demonstrated. However, one additional concern is the use of contrast agents; gadolinium compounds are known to cross the placenta and enter the fetal bloodstream, and it is recommended that their use be avoided. CT scans are performed more rapidly than MRI and therefore have less movement artefact.

The Department of Health identifies that patients need to understand in broad terms the nature and purpose of the procedure in order to give valid consent.

Within the maternity service responsibility for the coordination of information has been delegated to a group or an individual (patient information group).

Guidance should therefore emphasize the need to include:

- the risks associated with the proposed treatment
- the benefits of the proposed treatment
- the consequences of treatment
- alternative treatments available, and associated risks and benefits
- the consequences of not accepting the proposed treatment

100a. True
100b. True
100c. True
100d. False
100e. True – 1% miscarriage rate.

Note
Amniocentesis is used for prenatal diagnosis (e.g. Down syndrome) and is performed transabdominally from 15 weeks of gestation (amniotic fluid is aspirated through the abdominal wall). The procedure is performed under the guidance of ultrasonography to avoid injury to the fetus and placenta. Approximately 20–30 mL of fluid is withdrawn with a syringe attached to a needle (which is inserted into the amniotic fluid via the abdominal route). Cytogenetic and biochemical tests are carried out on amniocytes present in the amniotic fluid.

101a. False – is associated with limb defect when performed before 9 weeks.
101b. True
101c. False – is used as a diagnostic test for Down syndrome.
101d. True
101e. True

102a. True
102b. False
102c. False
102d. True
102e. True

Note
First trimester ultrasound is also used for dating of pregnancy, detection of anomalies such as spina bifida, checking viability of the fetus, checking the number of fetuses (e.g. multiple pregnancy) and guidance in performing chorionic villus biopsy.

103a. True
103b. True
103c. True
103d. True
103e. True

Note
The conditions that can be diagnosed by ultrasonography include: spina bifida, anencephaly, gastroschisis, dextrocardia, ventriculomegaly, hydrops fetalis and polycystic kidneys.

104a. True
104b. False
104c. True – is trisomy 18.
104d. False
104e. True – is trisomy 13.

Note
For a given species chromosomal number is fixed (diploid number in somatic cells is 46 while haploid is 23). In most cases non-dysjunction during meiosis (I or II) or mitosis is the main reason for aberrations in chromosomal number. Clinical syndromes can be caused by aberrations in both autosomal (e.g. trisomy 13, 18 and 21) and sex chromosomes, e.g. Turner syndrome (45XO), Klinefelter syndrome (47XXY) and triple X syndrome (47XXX).

105a. False– they are phenotypically males and show the presence of sex chromatin.
105b. True – the error during gametogenesis can occur during either first or second meiotic division or during both meiotic divisions.
105c. True
105d. False – the error during gametogenesis is maternal in most cases (64%) and paternal in the rest of the cases.
105e. False – 80–90% of all patients with this syndrome have a karyotype 47XXY and in the remaining 10% mosaicism is seen.

106a. True
106b. True
106c. True
106d. True
106e. False – single palmar or simian crease is seen in Down syndrome.

Note
The other features of Turner syndrome are cubitus valgus, short metacarpals, webbed neck, shield chest, ventricular septal defect, horseshoe kidney, pigmented naevi, lymphoedema of the hands and feet, and telangiectasis.

107a. True
107b. True
107c. False – it is due to an inborn error in purine and pyrimidine metabolism.
107d. True
107e. False – it is due to an inborn error in lipid metabolism.

108a. False – it is an autosomal recessive condition.
108b. True – onset of disease is 4–6 months.
108c. True
108d. True – also associated with physical growth retardation.
108e. False – is associated with hexosaminidase A deficiency and absence of this enzyme is seen in amniotic fluid cell cultures.

109a. False – it is an autosomal recessive condition.
109b. True – due to increased deposition of copper in the liver.
109c. True
109d. False – serum ceruloplasmin levels are very low. Serum copper is also low with high urinary copper levels.
109e. False – a Kayser–Fleischer ring is seen in the cornea.

Note
Wilson disease is an autosomal recessive condition in which there is accumulation of copper in the tissues. The clinical manifestation can vary depending on the copper deposition in various organs and mainly presents with liver, neurological or psychiatric symptoms and signs. The treatment includes a diet with low copper content (chocolates, mushrooms, dried fruits, shellfish and liver) and medication that increases its excretion or decreases its absorption, e.g. penicillamine causes chelation of copper and promotes its excretion in the urine.

110a. True
110b. False
110c. True
110d. True
110e. False – α-chain in HbS is same as normal haemoglobin (HbA). Glutamine is replaced by valine at the sixth amino acid position from the N-terminal end in the β-chain (HbS).

111a. False – they contain four γ-chains.
111b. False – they contain four β-chains.
111c. False – in haemoglobin C, glutamic acid is replaced by lysine at the sixth amino acid position from N-terminal end in the β-chain.
111d. True – haemoglobin A is also made of two α- and two β-chains.
111e. True

112a. True
112b. False
112c. False – thalassaemia is due to decreased synthesis of a particular globulin chain and accumulation of either free α- or β-chains occurs in the red cell precursors depending on the type of thalassaemia (α-thalassaemia, β-thalassaemia, etc.).
112d. False – is associated with bone marrow hyperplasia and the anaemia is due to haemolysis.
112e. True

113a. True
113b. False – may show low-voltage QRS complexes.
113c. True
113d. True
113e. True

114a. True – this is detected by increased urinary methionine and homocysteine levels.
114b. True – this is detected by raised phenylalanine in the blood (Guthrie test is used to diagnose this condition). The treatment is a phenylalanine-free diet.
114c. True – this is caused by reduced enzyme activity or deficiency of the enzyme, galactose-1-phosphate uridyl transferase, and usually detected by raised levels of galactose in both urine and blood.
114d. True – this is detected by increased levels of cysteine in the urine.
114e. True – this is detected by increased histidine levels in the blood and urine.

115a. True – serum creatine kinase (CK) is also increased in Duchenne muscular dystrophy.
115b. False – reduced G6PD (glucose-6-phosphate dehydrogenase) in red cells is seen in G6PD deficiency.
115c. False – factor VIII is reduced in haemophilia A and factor IX is reduced in haemophilia B.
115d. False – serum phosphorus is decreased.
115e. True

116a. True
116b. True
116c. False
116d. True – as human red blood cells do not contain a nucleus, they lack chromosomal deoxyribonucleic acid (DNA). During the process of erythropoiesis, they also lose mitochondria. Thus they produce energy by anaerobic glycolysis of glucose, producing lactic acid.
116e. False

Note
Red blood cells (RBCs) are special cells that carry oxygen from the lungs to different tissues in the body. They have a lifespan of 120 days and are subsequently destroyed in the reticuloendothelial system. The proteins in the haemoglobin are broken down to be reused for synthesis of new proteins while iron is transported back to the plasma and bone marrow for synthesis of haemoglobin in RBCs. The porphyrin (red pigment) in the porphyrin ring structure of haemoglobin (where iron is attached) is converted to bilirubin (yellow pigment). Subsequent to its formation, bilirubin is then released into the plasma and transported to the liver, where it undergoes changes, to be secreted into the bile. The rate-limiting step in bilirubin formation is the degree or amount of haemoglobin destruction.

117a. True
117b. False
117c. True
117d. False
117e. True

Note
Calcitonin prevents bone resorption and cannot be given by the oral route. It can be given by either the nasal or the parenteral route. The nasal route is preferred even though absorption is slow. It causes nausea, vomiting, diarrhoea and hot flushes. It has been shown to reduce vertebral fractures and is less effective than bisphosphonates in the treatment of postmenopausal osteoporosis.

118a. True
118b. False – does not affect non-vertebral fractures.
118c. True
118d. True
118e. False – does not reduce the risk of coronary heart disease.

Note
There are three types of oestrogen (E) receptors: E_1, E_2 and E_3. SERMs have both agonist and antagonist actions on different sites on E_2 receptors.

119a. True
119b. False
119c. True
119d. True
119e. True

Note
Aminoglycosides inhibit translation (protein synthesis).

120a. True
120b. False
120c. True
120d. False
120e. True

Note
Three cycles of 30-minute intervals of boiling, followed by periods of cooling, kill bacterial endospores (intermittent boiling), whereas continuous boiling kills microbial pathogens and vegetative forms of bacteria but may not kill bacterial endospores.

121a. True
121b. True
121c. False
121d. True
121e. True

Note
MRSA strains are resistant to the action of meticillin and related β-lactam antibiotics (e.g. penicillin and cephalosporins).

122a. False
122b. True
122c. False
122d. True
122e. False

Note
HBV surface antigen is detectable in the bloodstream from 1 to 6 months after infection, but anti-HBsAg is detectable from only about 8 months. Because of the large amounts of HBV surface antigen that are not associated with infectious virus, the presence of HBeAg is the best marker for infectious virus. HBeAb suggests low risk of transmission, as it appears after the virus is not detectable in the bloodstream.

123a. True
123b. False – it is obtaining multiple copies of DNA, not RNA.
123c. True
123d. True
123e. False

124a. True
124b. True
124c. True
124d. False
124e. True

Note
A vector is an agent that can carry a DNA fragment into a host cell. This can multiply autonomously in the host-like bacteria and subsequently DNA is isolated in the pure form for analysis. This finally leads to production of many copies of the specific DNA sequence of interest.

125a. True
125b. True
125c. True
125d. False – it gives large quantities of pure DNA.
125e. True

Note
The main disadvantage can be contamination in the laboratory.

126a. False – it is composed of a single polynucleotide chain.
126b. True
126c. True – it is required for the formation of RNA chains from DNA templates.
126d. False – mRNA is produced in nucleus.
126e. True – ribosomal RNA (rRNA) is also involved in protein synthesis.

127a. False – in the UK, cervical cancer screening starts at the age of 25 years and women below the age of 20 years are not screened, as cervical cancer is rare and screening is thought to cause more harm than good.
127b. True
127c. True
127d. True
127e. True

128a. False – HPV type depends on DNA homology.
128b. True
128c. True
128d. True
128e. True

129a. True
129b. True – it is also associated with multinucleation and irregular nuclear margin (nuclear abnormalities are seen involving the whole thickness (two-thirds or more) of squamous epithelium with an intact basement membrane).
129c. False – pyknotic nuclei are seen in normal cells.
129d. False – this form of treatment is used in stage I cervical cancer.
129e. False – colposcopy is performed before any treatment. In cases of high-grade CIN either a see-and-treat policy can be adapted or a biopsy can be taken before arranging treatment. At present most units use LLETZ (large loop excision of the transformation zone) as the treatment procedure of choice unless there are any specific indications for doing a knife cone biopsy.

130a. False – LBC dramatically reduces the number of inadequate smears. Once the smear is taken, it is rinsed in the thin prep solution 10 times and is sent off to the laboratory. This sample is centrifuged to remove all other cell debris (lymphocytes), mucus and blood, which can cause problems in interpreting the smear (conventional smear). Subsequently the cells from the transformation zone are studied under the microscope after staining.
130b. True
130c. True
130d. True
130e. True

131a. False – CIN I is not an indication for knife cone biopsy of the cervix. It is an indication for further surveillance in the colposcopy clinic or for LLETZ if the abnormality persists or progresses.
131b. False – CIN II is an indication for LLETZ.
131c. False – HPV change in itself is not an indication for LLETZ as most of these changes regress or resolve by themselves. These women would need further surveillance with smear and colposcopy until a follow-up smear is normal.
131d. True
131e. True

132a. True – primary haemorrhage is also a complication.
132b. True
132c. True
132d. True
132e. False

133a. True
133b. True
133c. False
133d. False
133e. False

Note
The following are blood tests done at booking in low-risk women: FBC, blood group and antibody level, Hb electrophoresis to check for haemoglobinopathy, syphilis, hepatitis B, HIV testing and random blood sugar.

134a. True
134b. False – bleeding after 24 weeks due to premature separation of placenta before the delivery of the baby (abruption).
134c. True
134d. True
134e. False – anti-D is given only to women who are rhesus negative.

Note
The causes of APH include placenta praevia (major placenta praevia – placenta covering the cervical internal os – and minor placenta praevia – low lying or placenta situated within 2 cm of cervical internal os), abruption (revealed, concealed and mixed), local cervical causes (ectropion, cervical polyp and cervical cancer) and vasa praevia (fetal cause).

135a. True
135b. True
135c. False – pre-eclampsia is associated with intrauterine growth retardation (IUGR) due to placental insufficiency.
135d. True
135e. True

136a. False – liquor volume is decreased.
136b. False
136c. True – pulsatility index is also increased.
136d. True
136e. True

Note
In cases of placental insufficiency (blood flow to the fetus is decreased) there is asymmetrical IUGR (head sparing). In simple terms the baby is small due to starvation (degree might vary depending on the placental insufficiency).

In cases of genetic causes (chromosomal abnormalities), there is symmetrical IUGR. There can be associated abnormalities, which can be visualized by performing an ultrasound scan, but not always.

In cases of constitutionally small babies (depends on ethnicity, build of the mother and nutrition of the mother), the babies are normally small and do not have the features described above on ultrasound.

137a. False – it is the cervical length.
137b. True
137c. False – it is the position of the cervix (posterior, midline or anterior).
137d. True
137e. False – it is the station of the presenting part in relation to the ischial spines (above or below the spines).

138a. True
138b. True
138c. True
138d. True
138e. False – progesterone suppresses uterine activity by blocking the formation of oxytocin receptors and also gap junctions. Oxytocin receptors and gap junctions are required for initiation of uterine activity or contractions and also help the synchronization of uterine activity during labour.

139a. True
139b. False
139c. True
139d. False
139e. False

Note
The formation of oxytocin receptors and the gap junction is promoted by oestrogen.

140a. True
140b. True
140c. True
140d. False – the contractions are stronger in the upper segment of the uterus and become weaker towards the lower segment.
140e. True

141a. True – Secreted from supraoptic and paraventricular nuclei of the hypothalamus and stored in Herring bodies at axon terminals in the posterior pituitary.
141b. False – it is stored in the posterior lobe of the pituitary gland until required.
141c. True
141d. False – it is secreted in a pulsatile fashion in late pregnancy.
141e. True – the neuronal stimuli caused by distension of the cervix by the presenting part increase the secretion of oxytocin more frequently during labour. This is known as the Ferguson reflex.

142a. True
142b. True
142c. True
142d. False
142e. False – there is a decrease in sex hormone-binding globulin (SHBG).

143a. False – only 58% of women receive medical treatment before referral to a specialist.
143b. True
143c. False – in at least half of those who have a hysterectomy, menorrhagia is the main presenting problem.
143d. True
143e. True – it can interfere with physical, social and emotional quality of life.

Note
NICE guidelines published in January 2007 for heavy menstrual bleeding (HMB).

Reference:
National Collaborating Centre for Women's and Children's Health. *Heavy Menstrual Bleeding: Clinical guideline*. London: RCOG Press, 2007. Available at: www.nice.org.uk/CG044.

144a. True
144b. False – it is used in the treatment of fibroids causing menorrhagia.
144c. False – it is used in the treatment of fibroids causing menorrhagia.
144d. True
144e. True

145a. True
145b. True
145c. False – hypothyroidism can cause menorrhagia.
145d. True
145e. False – submucous and intramural fibroids can cause menorrhagia.

146a. True
146b. True
146c. True – HELLP – haemolysis, elevated liver enzymes and low platelets.
146d. True
146e. False

Note
The other causes of thrombocytopenia during pregnancy include gestational thrombocytopenia, immune thrombocytopenic purpura, severe pre-eclampsia, antiphospholipid antibody syndrome, thrombotic thrombocytopenic purpura and HIV infection.

Laboratory error should be ruled out by repeating the platelet count and also requesting a blood film to re-check the platelet count.

147a. True
147b. False – FDPs are increased.
147c. True
147d. False – PT is increased.
147e. True

Note
DIC is associated with consumption of the platelets and coagulation factors. As a result the fibrinolytic pathway is stimulated leading to increase in the FDPs. The platelet count and coagulation factors in the blood are decreased but clotting times are increased.

The causes of DIC during pregnancy include: severe pre-eclampsia, HELLP syndrome, abruption, amniotic fluid embolism, massive postpartum haemorrhage, chorioamnionitis and septic miscarriage or abortion.

The treatment depends on the underlying cause and also replacement of red blood cells and coagulation factors (fresh frozen plasma, cryoprecipitate and platelet concentrates).

148a. False – von Willebrand factor (vWf) and factor VIII may be reduced; vWf is required for the stability of factor VIII and platelet function.
148b. False – clotting time is prolonged in haemophilia.
148c. True
148d. True
148e. True – therefore there is an increased risk of primary and secondary postpartum haemorrhage.

149a. False
149b. True – schistocytes (red cell fragments) are seen on blood film.
149c. True – irritability, drowsiness, headache, seizures and coma.
149d. False
149e. True

Note
- TTP is also characterized by a raised temperature or fever.
- The unconjugated bilurubin is increased depending on the degree of anaemia.
- The lactate dehydrogenase is also increased.
- The clotting time and fibrinogen concentrations are normal, unlike DIC.

150a. True – it is a protozoan infection caused by *Plasmodium falciparum*, *P. vivax*, *P. malariae* and *P. ovale*.
150b. True
150c. False – it increases the risk of premature labour and second trimester miscarriage.
150d. False – it usually causes decrease in birth weight of the baby.
150e. True

151a. True – it recurs in subsequent pregnancy.
151b. False – is associated with abnormal liver function tests and electrolytes due to vomiting and dehydration.
151c. True
151d. True – Mallory–Weiss tear is a tear in the mucosa at the junction of the stomach and the oesophagus. It causes bleeding resulting in haematemesis.
151e. True – severe hyperemesis gravidarum can cause a deficiency of thiamine (vitamin B_1) resulting in Wernicke encephalopathy. It is characterized by confusion, diplopia, ataxia and ophthalmoplegia (sixth nerve palsy and nystagmus).

152a. True
152b. False – metabolic rate is increased by 20%.
152c. True
152d. True
152e. False – There is rise in arterial PO_2 and fall in arterial PCO_2 due to hyperventilation resulting in a fall in serum bicarbonate (compensated respiratory alkalosis is normal during pregnancy).

153a. True
153b. True
153c. True
153d. True
153e. True

Note
Suggested reading: RCOG. *Green-top Guideline No. 28. Thromboembolic disease in pregnancy and the puerperium: acute management*. London: RCOG, 2007.

154a. True
154b. True
154c. False – pleural effusion may be seen.
154d. False
154e. True

155a. True
155b. False
155c. True
155d. False
155e. False

Note
Suggested reading: RCOG. *Green-top Guideline No. 28. Thromboembolic disease in pregnancy and the puerperium: acute management.* London: RCOG, 2007.

156a. False – the most common autoantibody is antinuclear antibody (ANA).
156b. False – these are the most specific antibodies.
156c. False – both antibodies cross the placenta. These antibodies are directed against cytoplasmic ribonucleoproteins and can cause transient cutaneous lupus and congenital heart block in neonates.
156d. False – glomerulonephritis occurs more frequently in women with these autoantibodies.
156e. False – ANA is seen in 96% of SLE patients.

157a. True
157b. True
157c. True
157d. True
157e. True

Note
The other causes of seizures during pregnancy include: epilepsy, hypoglycaemia (diabetes), hypocalcaemia (magnesium sulphate therapy), hyponatraemia (hyperemesis), space-occupying lesion and pseudo-epilepsy.

158a. False – is caused by IgG antibodies (also blocks the neuromuscular transmission).
158b. False – is associated with weakness and fatigue of striated muscle.
158c. True – is also associated with dysphagia and thymoma in 10% of the patients.
158d. True – lack of fetal movement causing fetal contractures (this is due to transplacental transfer of antibodies).
158e. False – edrophonium chloride (short-acting anticholinesterase) is administered to make a diagnosis of myasthenia gravis (basis of Tensilon test – transient improvement in the muscle strength is observed).

159a. True – the IgG antibodies bind to the basement membrane in the skin, evoking an immune response leading to formation of subepidermal vesicles. Also seen is complement (C3) deposition at the basement membrane zone, demonstrated by direct immunofluorescence on skin biopsy specimen (this test is used for diagnosis along with clinical features).
159b. False – is rare during pregnancy.
159c. False – require treatment with topical steroids and most require systemic steroids.
159d. True
159e. True – the skin lesions (intensely pruritic) start around the umbilicus and then spread to the periphery (limbs, palms and soles).

160a. True
160b. True
160c. True
160d. True
160e. True

Note
The other causes of acute renal failure during pregnancy include massive postpartum haemorrhage, septic abortion, bilateral ureteric damage or obstruction, and severe hyperemesis gravidarum.

161a. False – most women are usually asymptomatic (95%) and 50–60% of women in the UK are already immune due to previous subclinical infection.
161b. False – the primary infection occurs in approximately 1–2% of pregnant women. The anti-CMV IgM antibodies are increased during primary infection and disappear by 4–8 months after primary infection.
161c. True
161d. False – if the mother is infected, fetal damage occurs in about 4% (this means that most infected fetuses are not affected). It also accounts for approximately 10% of learning disabilities in children aged 6 years and below.
161e. False – recurrent CMV is rarely associated with fetal damage.

Note
The cytomegalovirus belongs to the herpes family. It can cause congenital infection (this occurs when the mother suffers primary infection or reactivation during pregnancy) and also life-threatening infections in patients who are immunocompromised (e.g. patients with a kidney transplant and HIV).

In adults, it presents with non-specific symptoms such as fever and malaise and is associated with lymphadenopathy. The various routes of its transmission include blood transfusion and transplantation. In temperate countries, infection is usually transmitted by close or sexual contact and approximately 1–2% of the population is affected in this way each year.

Effects on the fetus and clinical manifestations in the newborn can include: chorioretinitis, microcephaly, intracranial calcification, hepatosplenomegaly, jaundice, thrombocytopenia and intrauterine growth retardation.

162a. False
162b. False
162c. True – hepatitis E is a non-enveloped, single-stranded RNA virus and is transmitted via the faecal-oral route (contaminated water and food). It is more common in countries with poor sanitation and can cause an epidemic outbreak. Generally it is a self-limiting infection but fulminant hepatitis is more common in pregnant women and is associated with a mortality rate of 20%.
162d. True – Primary varicella infection during pregnancy can cause serious maternal morbidity (pneumonia (10%), hepatitis and encephalitis) and mortality (case fatality rate of less than 1%).

Reference: Royal College of Obstetricians and Gynaecologists. *Green-top Guideline No. 13. Chickenpox in pregnancy.* London: Royal College of Obstetricians and Gynaecologists, 2007. Available at: www.rcog.org.uk/files/rcog-corp/uploaded-files/GT13ChickenpoxinPregnancy2007.pdf.

162e. True

163a. False
163b. True
163c. False
163d. False – infection may be transmitted to the fetus *in utero*.
163e. True

164a. False – it is a motile Gram-positive bacterium.
164b. True
164c. True
164d. False – 70% of the healthy population carry this organism.
164e. True – postmortem examinations of infected neonates also show the same finding.

165a. False
164b. True
165c. False
165d. False
165e. True

Note

Mumps is an acute generalized infection of children and young adults, caused by a paramyxovirus. The incubation period is between 14 and 18 days. It spreads by close contact and by droplets. The swelling of the face is the most common symptom (parotitis). Clinically it can manifest as meningitis, orchitis and oophoritis. Vaccination of susceptible individuals is the mainstay of prevention.

166a. True – endothelial stem cells can be obtained from the placenta.
166b. True
166c. True – haematopoietic, mesenchymal and endothelial stem cells can be obtained from the bone marrow.
166d. True – haematopoietic, epithelial and mesenchymal stem cells can be obtained from the liver.
166e. True

Note
Fetal stem cells can be obtained from fetal tissues such as kidneys (mesenchymal stem cell), lungs (mesenchymal stem cell), pancreas (mesenchymal and epithelial stem cell), brain and spinal cord (neural stem cell).

167a. True
167b. False – cord blood requires less strict criteria for tissue type matching between potential recipient and donor than required for bone marrow donors.
167c. False – cord blood recipients have been shown to have less severe graft-versus-host reaction than bone marrow recipients.
167d. True
167e. True

168a. False – during the first half of pregnancy, most of the amniotic fluid is obtained from active sodium and potassium transport across the amniotic membrane and fetal skin.
168b. False
168c. False – in addition to fetal urine, a major source of amniotic fluid is also obtained from the respiratory tract.
168d. False – only a minor amount is obtained from fetal swallowing and the gastrointestinal tract.
168e. False – most of the amniotic fluid is obtained from fetal micturition (fetal urine).

169a. False
169b. True
169c. False – causes decrease in the proportion of women with blood loss of 500 mL or more.
169d. False
169e. True

Note
Active management of the third stage of labour is delivery of the placenta by using uterotonic drugs plus controlled cord traction. The various drugs that are used include oxytocin, oxytocin–ergometrine combination, ergometrine and prostaglandins.

170a. True
170b. True
170c. True

170d. True
170e. True

Note
APS is an autoimmune disorder that can cause thrombosis, fetal loss (miscarriage or stillbirth) and early onset severe pre-eclampsia. In the absence of other associated diseases it is called primary APS and in the presence of associated autoimmune diseases (e.g. SLE) it is called secondary APS. It is characterized by formation of antibodies against cardiolipin and β_2-glycoprotein I and lupus anticoagulant, which forms the basis of a blood test for its diagnosis (done twice at an interval of 3 months to confirm the results). It can also give a false-positive test for syphilis.

171a. False – the use of the wrong management plan to achieve an aim or failure of an action to be completed as intended.
171b. True
171c. False – an injury caused by medical management and not by the underlying condition or disease.
171d. True
171e. True

172a. True
172b. True
172c. True
172d. True
172e. True

Note
The other pillars of clinical governance include: using information and IT, staff and staffing management (making seven pillars in all).

173a. True
173b. True
173c. True
173d. True
173e. True

174a. False – the CNST management programme started in 1996.
174b. True
174c. True
174d. True
174e. True

175a. True
175b. True
175c. False – macroprolactinomas are associated with values $>$5000 mU/L.
175d. True

175e. False – drug therapy (cabergoline and bromocriptine) is the first line unless causing any intracranial pressure symptoms.

Note

Prolactin is a peptide hormone and structurally similar to growth hormone. It is mainly under inhibitory control of hypothalamus. It follows a circadian rhythm with the highest plasma concentration during sleep. Dopamine inhibits prolactin secretion and is provided by dopaminergic neurons of the periventricular and arcuate nuclei of the medial basal hypothalamus. It reaches the pituitary gland through the hypothalamic–hypophyseal–portal system.

The physiological causes of raised prolactin are pregnancy, lactation, breast stimulation, stress, sexual intercourse and exercise.

The hormones that promote prolactin secretion are thyrotrophin-releasing hormone, oxytocin, vasopressin and vasoactive intestinal peptide.

The drugs causing hyperprolactinaemia include phenothiazines, haloperidol, metoclopramide, methyldopa, morphine, methadone, oestrogens, cocaine and cimetidine.

Prolactin values >5000 mU/L are typically seen in macroprolactinomas.

Hyperprolactinaemia can present as oligo-/amenorrhoea, infertility, galactorrhoea and decreased libido. It can cause a decrease in bone density in both men and women. Mass effects such as headache, visual field defects and cranial nerve palsies can be seen with pituitary macroprolactinomas.

Dopamine agonists have a major role in the management of hyperprolactinaemia. The three drugs that are licensed in the UK are bromocriptine, cabergoline and quinagolide.

3. Practice EMQs I: Questions

1–4)

Options

A.	Alchohol
B.	Amiodarone
C.	ACE inhibitors
D.	Diethylstilbestrol
E.	Isotretinoin
F.	Streptomycin
G.	Sodium valproate
H.	Thalidomide
I.	Radioactive iodine

Instructions: Select the most likely teratogenic agent from the list of options above for the fetal abnormalities mentioned below. Each option may be used once, more than once or not at all.

1) Thymic aplasia

2) Limb defects

3) Vaginal adenosis

4) Deafness

5–8)

Options

A.	Clindamycin
B.	Chloramphenicol
C.	Erythromycin
D.	Metronidazole
E.	Nitrofurantoin
F.	Tetracycline
G.	Tobramycin
H.	Streptomycin
I.	Sulfadiazine
J.	Sulfamethoxazole

Instructions: Select the likely drug from the list of options above for the side effects mentioned below. Each option may be used once, more than once or not at all.

5) Aplastic anaemia

6) Cholestatic jaundice

7) Grey baby syndrome

8) Discoloration of the teeth

9–12)

Options

A.	Interleukin 1
B.	Interleukin 2
C.	Interleukin 4
D.	Interleukin 5
E.	Interleukin 6
F.	Interleukin 10
G.	Interleukin 11
H.	Interleukin 12
I.	Interferon-α
J.	Transforming growth factor-β

Instructions: Select the most appropriate cytokines for each of the actions referred to below from the list of options above. Each option may be used once, more than once or not at all.

9) Promotes the resistance of cells to viral infection

10) Causes the activation of T cells and macrophages

11) Promotes the growth of B cells and eosinophils

12) Promotes B-cell growth and antibody production

13–16)

Options

A.	Alveolar ventilation
B.	Expiratory reserve volume
C.	Functional residual capacity
D.	Inspiratory reserve volume
E.	Minute volume
F.	Residual volume
G.	Tidal volume
H.	Total lung capacity
I.	Total alveolar capacity
J.	Vital capacity

Instructions: Select the most appropriate lung volume for each of the definitions referred to below from the list of options above. Each option may be used once, more than once or not at all.

13) The volume of air in the lungs after maximal expiration

14) The volume of air inspired in a minute

15) The volume of air in the lungs after maximal inspiration

16) Tidal volume minus dead space volume

17–20)

Options

A.	Acute myocardial infarction
B.	Atrial fibrillation
C.	Complete heart block
D.	Hyperkalaemia
E.	Hypokalaemia
F.	Left bundle-branch block
G.	Pulmonary embolism
H.	Right bundle-branch block
I.	Ventricular bigemini
J.	Wolff–Parkinson–White syndrome

Instructions: Select the most appropriate cardiovascular condition from the above list of options for each case described below. Each option may be used once, more than once or not at all.

17) A 25-year-old woman who is 30 weeks pregnant attends A&E with shortness of breath. Her electrocardiogram (ECG) shows tachycardia and S1Q3T3 pattern (S wave in lead 1, Q wave in lead 3, inverted T wave in lead 3).

18) A 60-year-old woman, who underwent a hysterectomy 4 days ago, complains of an inability to pass much urine and her ECG is showing tall T waves.

19) A 35-year-old woman who is 28 weeks pregnant comes to the day assessment unit with a history of palpitations. Her ECG shows a short P–R interval, slurring of the upstroke of QRS complex (delta wave) and wide QRS complexes.

20) A 45-year-old morbidly obese woman comes to A&E with a history of central chest pain and shortness of breath. She is 20 weeks pregnant and her ECG shows ST elevation in leads V1 to V4.

21–24)

Options

A.	Limb hypoplasia
B.	Microphthalmia
C.	Neural tube defect
D.	Cataract
E.	Malformed uterus
F.	Mandibular hypoplasia
G.	Maxillary hypoplasia
H.	Chondrodysplasia
I.	Gastroschisis
J.	Cleft palate

Instructions: Select the most appropriate congenital malformations above for each of the teratogens referred to below. Each option may be used once, more than once or not at all.

21) Alchohol

22) Diethylstilbestrol (DES)

23) Cocaine

24) Isotretinoin

25–28)

Options

A.	Bulla
B.	Ecchymosis
C.	Macule
D.	Nodule
E.	Papule
F.	Petechia
G.	Purpura
H.	Pustule
I.	Ulcer
J.	Vesicle

Instructions: Select the most appropriate skin lesions from the list of options for each of the morphological descriptions referred to below. Each option may be used once, more than once or not at all.

25) Large papule (>0.5 cm)

26) Yellowish-white pus-filled lesion

27) A small fluid-filled blister

28) A large fluid-filled blister

29–32)

Options

A.	Atrophic endometrium
B.	Chronic endometritis
C.	Complex hyperplasia with atypia
D.	Complex hyperplasia without atypia
E.	Endometrial adenocarcinoma
F.	Exogenous progesterone effect
G.	Endometrial changes in follicular phase
H.	Endometrial changes in luteal phase
I.	Plasma cell endometritis
J.	Simple hyperplasia

Instructions: Select the most appropriate diagnosis for the list of options above for the following endometrial changes given below. Each option may be used once, more than once or not at all.

29) Endometrial glands are elongated with a narrow lumen and dense surrounding stroma. The spiral arteries elongate and span the length of the endometrium

30) Endometrial glands are tortuous with a large lumen secreting glycogen and mucus. The spiral arteries extend into the superficial layer of the endometrium

31) Cystic dilated glands of variable size with crowding and budding of the glands. The stroma between adjacent glands is reduced

32) Cystic dilated glands of variable size with gland cells showing cell stratification, tufting, loss of nuclear polarity, enlarged nuclei and increase in mitotic activity. There is no invasion into the connective tissue

33–36)

Options

A.	Anencephaly
B.	Arnold–Chiari malformation
C.	Choroid plexus cysts
D.	Encephalocele
E.	Holoprosencephaly
F.	Hydranencephaly
G.	Miller–Dieker syndrome
H.	Spina bifida occulta
I.	Sacrococcygeal teratoma
J.	Schizencephaly
K.	Walker–Warburg syndrome

Instructions: Match the ultrasound findings described below with the list of diagnoses mentioned above. Each option may be used once, more than once or not at all.

33) Absence of the cranial vault and cerebral hemispheres

34) Protrusion of the cranial structures through a calvarial bone defect

35) A large solid/cystic mass arising from sacrococcygeal area associated with polyhydramnios and hydrops in the fetus

36) A large fluid collection filling the whole cranial cavity, replacing the normal brain tissue

37–40)

Options

A.	Choriocarcinoma
B.	Dysgerminoma
C.	Embryonal carcinoma
D.	Endodermal sinus tumour
E.	Granulosa cell tumour
F.	Immature teratoma
G.	Mature teratoma
H.	Serous cystadenocarcinoma
I.	Theca cell tumour
J.	Sertoli–Leydig cell tumour

Instructions: Match the most appropriate ovarian tumour mentioned above with their respective tumour markers/hormones given below. Each option may be used once, more than once or not at all.

37) Inhibin

38) Lactate dehydrogenase

39) α-Fetoprotein

40) Oestrogen

41–44)

Options

A.	*Coxiella burnetii*
B.	*Donovania granulomatis*
C.	*Haemophilus ducreyi*
D.	*Rickettsia typhi*
E.	*Rickettsia conorii*
F.	*Rickettsia rickettsii*
G.	*Rickettsia prowazekii*
H.	*Sarcoptes scabiei*
I.	*Trypanosoma cruzi*
J.	*Treponema pallidum*

Instructions: Select the single most likely organism from the list of options above for each of the diseases mentioned below. Each option may be used once, more than once or not at all.

41) Rocky Mountain spotted fever

42) Q fever

43) Epidemic typhus

44) Murine typhus

45–48)

Options

A.	*Trichomonas vaginalis* (TV)
B.	*Candida albicans*
C.	Human papillomavirus
D.	Herpes simplex virus
E.	*Treponema pallidum*
F.	Bacterial vaginosis (BV)
G.	*Chlamydia trachomatis*
H.	*Haemophilus ducreyi*
I.	*Neisseria gonorrhoeae*
J.	Lymphogranuloma venereum

Instructions: For each case described below, choose the single most likely cause of infection from the list of options above. Each option may be used once, more than once or not at all.

45) A 36-year-old woman presents to the sexual heath clinic with an offensive creamy yellow vaginal discharge. A saline wet mount of the discharge under microscope revealed motile, flagellated protozoa

46) A 20-year-old woman presents to the sexual health clinic with a grey–white offensive homogeneous vaginal discharge. Microscopy of the discharge revealed clue cells with a positive whiff test

47) A 30-year-old woman presents with pain on urination and intercourse. She has travelled abroad recently. On examination, she has tender vulval ulcers with buboes in the inguinal region

48) A 17-year-old girl presents to the GUM clinic with an offensive vaginal discharge and dysuria. Gram staining shows intracellular bean-shaped diplococci

49–52)

Options

A.	Appearance of a primitive streak
B.	Heart is prominent and circulation is established
C.	Ossification centres are apparent
D.	Pigmentation of the retina
E.	Appearance of upper limb buds
F.	Formation of digits and eyelids
G.	Appearance of hind limb buds, otic vesicle and lens placode
H.	Herniation of the bowel through the umbilicus is prominent
I.	Protrusion of allantois into the body stalk
J.	Formation of the notochord from the blastophore

Instructions: Match the most appropriate event during the embryonic period from the list of options above with the period in days post-conception given below. Each option may be used once, more than once or not at all.

49) 14–15 days post-conception

50) 28–30 days post-conception

51) 21–28 days post-conception

52) 26–27 days post-conception

53–56)

Options

A.	Anorexia nervosa
B.	Bulimia nervosa
C.	Cryptomenorrhoea
D.	Hypothalamic amenorrhoea
E.	Hyperprolactinaemia
F.	Hypothyroidism
G.	Hyperthyroidism
H.	Menopause
I.	Polycystic ovarian syndrome (PCOS)
J.	Pregnancy

Instructions: For each case described below, choose the single most likely cause of amenorrhoea from the list of options above. Each option may be used once more than once or not at all.

53) A 30-year-old woman with BMI of 40 presents to the gynaecology outpatient clinic with irregular periods and hirsutism. She also gives a history of recent-onset hypertension and type 2 diabetes. Clinically there are no signs of virilism

54) A 35-year-old woman presents to the gynaecology outpatient clinic with a 1-year history of amenorrhoea and secondary infertility. She has been taking haloperidol daily for the past 2 years and is known to suffer from schizophrenia. Previously she had a history of regular periods

55) A 14-year-old girl is brought by her mother to the outpatient clinic as she has not started menstruating. On further questioning, the daughter gives a history of cyclical lower abdominal pain every month for the previous 6 months

56) A 48-year-old woman complains of hot flushes, night sweats and no periods for the last 14 months. Her serum FSH is 52 IU/L. She is known to suffer from multiple sclerosis and gives a history of incontinence for the last 6 months

57–60)

Options

A.	Anorexia nervosa
B.	Asherman syndrome
C.	Cryptamenorrhoea
D.	Hypothalamic amenorrhoea
E.	Post-pill amenorrhoea
F.	Premature ovarian failure
G.	Pituitary microprolactinoma
H.	Pituitary macroprolactinoma
I.	Rokitansky–Küster–Hauser syndrome
J.	Sheehan syndrome

Instructions: For each case described below, choose the single most likely cause of primary and secondary amenorrhoea from the list of options above. Each option may be used once more than once or not at all.

57) A 16-year-old girl is referred to the gynaecology outpatient clinic by her general practitioner. On clinical examination, she has a small blind-ending vagina with normal development of secondary sexual characters. The ultrasound scan shows follicles in the right and left ovaries with an absent uterus

58) A 26-year-old woman presents to her general practitioner with a 6-month history of amenorrhoea after the delivery of her baby. She also complains of lethargy, somnolescence and weight gain. She is bottle feeding her baby as she was unable to produce breast milk. Her urine pregnancy test is negative. She had a postpartum haemorrhage of three litres after the delivery

59) A general practitioner refers a 31-year-old woman to the gynaecology outpatient clinic with a 12-month history of amenorrhoea. She had been on the combined pill for the last 10 years, which she stopped 6 months ago as she is trying to conceive. Her blood test result shows FSH (follicle-stimulating hormone) 70 IU/L and LH (luteinizing hormone) 50 IU/L. Her urine pregnancy test is negative

60) A 26-year-old woman gives a 6-month history of amenorrhoea. She had two first trimester terminations in the past and also had an evacuation of retained products of conception for an incomplete miscarriage 6 months ago. Her hormonal studies show that she is ovulating and her urine pregnancy test is negative

61–64)

Options

A.	Adenovirus
B.	Cytomegalovirus
C.	Epstein–Barr virus
D.	Herpes simplex virus type 1
E.	Human papillomavirus types 1 and 4
F.	Human immunodeficiency virus
G.	Hepatitis B virus
H.	Human papillomavirus types 6 and 11
I.	Human papillomavirus types 16, 18, 31 and 33
J.	Varicella-zoster virus

Instructions: Select the single most likely viral infective organism from the list of options above for each case described below. Each option may be used once, more than once or not at all.

61) A 35-year-old woman is seen in the colposcopy clinic for a referral smear of moderate dyskaryosis. Colposcopy revealed a dense acetowhite area on acetic acid application suggestive of CIN III (cervical intraepithelial neoplasia III)

62) A 25-year-old woman presented to the sexual health clinic as she noticed multiple small bumps on her vulva. Clinical examination revealed warty lesions in both vulval and perianal regions

63) A 26-year-old woman attends the sexual health clinic with painful itchy sores on the perineum with an ulcer on the lower lip. She went on a holiday to Amsterdam and returned back 7 days ago. She gives a history of engaging in both vaginal and oral sex

64) A 14-year-old girl is admitted to the emergency medical ward with severe malaise, low-grade fever, pharyngitis and cervical lymphadenopathy. The monospot blood test is positive and the blood film shows monocytosis

65–68)

Options

A.	Bladder
B.	Ectocervix
C.	Endocervix
D.	Fallopian tube
E.	Labia majora
F.	Bartholin gland
G.	Skin of vestibule
H.	Ovarian surface
I.	Uterus
J.	Vagina

Instructions: Select the single most appropriate genital/pelvic organ from the above list of options for the epithelial linings described below. Each option may be used once, more than once or not at all.

65) Transitional epithelium

66) Keratinized stratified squamous epithelium with hair follicles

67) Stratified squamous epithelium without hair follicles

68) Non-keratinized stratified squamous epithelium

69–72)

Options

A.	Coeliac trunk
B.	Inferior phrenic artery
C.	Inferior mesenteric artery
D.	Lumbar artery
E.	Median sacral artery
F.	Middle suprarenal artery
G.	Ovarian artery
H.	Renal artery
I.	Superior mesenteric artery

Instructions: Select the single most appropriate branch of the aorta from the list of options above with the blood supply of the organs below. Each option may be used once, more than once or not at all.

69) Lateral branch of aorta supplying the diaphragm

70) Dorsal branch of aorta supplying the sacrum

71) Ventral branch of aorta supplying the gallbladder, pancreas and spleen

72) Ventral branch of aorta supplying the bowel from the transverse colon to the rectum

73–76)

Options

A.	Blood and body fluids
B.	Contact with lesions
C.	Contact with cat litter
D.	Dairy products
E.	Direct contact with respiratory secretions
F.	Faeco-oral
G.	Infected water
H.	Mosquito bite
I.	Sharing needles
J.	Uncooked meat

Instructions: Select the most appropriate route of transmission from the list of options above for each virus described below. Each option may be used once, more than once or not at all.

73) Hepatitis E virus

74) Hepatitis A virus

75) Respiratory syncytial virus

76) Cytomegalovirus

77–80)

Options

A.	Anterior paraventricular nucleus
B.	Arcuate nucleus
C.	Lateral and superior paraventricular nucleus
D.	Lateral and superior paraventricular nucleus and supraoptic nuclei
E.	Median paraventricular nucleus
F.	Preoptic area
G.	Periventricular area
H.	Hypothalamus
I.	Thalamus
J.	Anterior pituitary

Instructions: Match the most appropriate secreting area in the brain from the above list of options with the hormones mentioned below. Each option may be used once, more than once or not at all.

77) Vasopressin

78) Oxytocin

79) Thyrotrophin-releasing hormone

80) Corticotrophin-releasing hormone

3. Practice EMQs I: Answers

1) **E**

2) **H**

3) **D**

4) **F**

Note

Pharmaceutical risk categories used by the FDA (Food and Drug Administration)

Category A: controlled trials in humans have not shown fetal risk during the first trimester (and there is no evidence of risk during the second half of the pregnancy); the possibility of damage to the fetus appears remote.

Category B: animal studies during reproduction have not demonstrated risk to the fetus and controlled trials in humans do not exist (there is no confirmed evidence of damage during the first trimester or during the advanced stages of pregnancy).

Category C: animal studies have shown damaging effects on the fetus (teratogenic, lethal or other) and controlled trials have not been performed in women. The drug should be prescribed only if the potential benefit justifies and outweighs the risk to the fetus.

Category D: there is evidence of fetal risk in humans, but these drugs are used if the benefits of use during pregnancy for maternal indications (e.g. severe illness) outweigh the risk to the fetus.

Category X: animal and human studies have shown fetal anomalies. The risks of using these drugs during pregnancy outweigh the benefits. Therefore these drugs are contraindicated in pregnant women or in women who may intend to become pregnant.

Drugs and teratogenicity

Alchohol: fetal alcohol syndrome is caused by excessive maternal consumption of alcohol during pregnancy. It is associated with a short philtrum, thin vermillion and small palpebral fissures. The full range of disabilities that may arise from increased maternal consumption of alchohol is now described as fetal alcohol spectrum disorder (FASD).

Amiodarone: it is an antiarrhythmic agent used for treatment of ventricular and supraventricular arrhythmias. It is metabolized in the liver. It can be associated with interstitial lung disease, abnormal thyroid function tests, symptoms of hypothyroidism and hyperthyroidism (amiodarone contains 37% iodine by weight and its structure resembles thyroxine), and abnormal liver function tests, and rarely causes hepatitis and jaundice. Due to its iodine content, iodine overload is proposed to cause persistent inhibition of fetal thyroid function, leading to hypothyroidism and goitre.

ACE inhibitors: the use of these drugs in the second half of the pregnancy is known to cause fetal growth retardation, renal damage, oligohydramnios, pulmonary hypoplasia, hypocalvaria (cranial ossification defects), neonatal renal failure and death.

Diethylstilbestrol (DES): it is a non-steroidal oestrogen and was used for treating menopausal symptoms, prevention of miscarriage and preterm birth in the past. Subsequently studies showed that *in utero* exposure to DES caused vaginal adenosis and vaginal clear cell adenocarcinoma in the female offspring. It is also known to cause genital tract abnormalities (T-shaped uterus, transverse vaginal and cervical ridges) and infertility.

Streptomycin: eighth cranial nerve damage and deafness can occur.

Thalidomide: it was withdrawn from the market after identification of limb defects in babies born to mothers exposed to this drug in the first trimester. It causes amelia, phocomelia, cardiac defects, deafness, learning disabilities and autism.

Radioactive iodine: can cause damage to the thyroid gland, hypothyroidism and learning disabilities.

Iodides and iodine: Exposure after the tenth week of pregnancy causes hypothyroidism and goitre in neonates.

5) B

6) C

7) B

8) F

Note
Antibiotics, uses and side effects

Clindamycin: it is used in the treatment of bacterial infections and can cause a serious condition of the bowel called pseudomembranous colitis (caused by *Clostridium difficile* and presents with symptoms such as abdominal cramps, persistent smelly diarrhoea and fever – may lead to toxic megacolon and death). This infection is treated with oral metronidazole or oral vancomycin and obviously clindamycin would need to be stopped.

Chloramphenicol: it can cause nausea, vomiting, diarrhoea, headache, grey baby syndrome in infants and rarely aplastic anaemia (can present with fever, chills, sore throat or being unwell).

Erythromycin: it is a macrolide antibiotic and is used in the treatment of acne, chlamydia infection, syphilis (in patients allergic to penicillin), Legionnaires disease, otitis media, pharyngitis and laryngitis.

The side effects include nausea, vomiting, abdominal pain, abnormal liver function tests, hepatitis and yellowish discoloration of the skin and eyes as well as allergic skin reactions. It is safe to use in pregnancy and lactation.

Metronidazole: it is used for treatment of anaerobic infections and certain parasitic infections, e.g. *Clostridium difficile*, *Helicobacter pylori* (used in combination with other drugs), *Trichomonas vaginalis*, bacterial vaginosis, *Gardnerella vaginalis* and *Giardia lamblia*. It is not used in the first trimester of pregnancy.

The side effects include nausea, headache, a metallic taste and loss of appetite. Alcohol intake should be avoided as it can cause severe vomiting, abdominal cramps, flushing and headache if taken with metronidazole.

Tetracycline: it causes photosensitivity. It is contraindicated during pregnancy (as there is a possibility of altering the normal dentition and deposition of the drug in the bone during the process of growth). The teeth can be discoloured (greyish brown) and vary according to the dosage and period of use.

Streptomycin: it is associated with ototoxicity and nephrotoxicity.

Sulfadiazine: it is a sulphonamide antibiotic and contraindicated in people who are sensitive to sulfa drugs. Several side affects including erythema multiforme (Stevens–Johnson syndrome), generalized skin eruptions, bone marrow depression, agranulocytosis, nausea, vomiting and abdominal cramps have been associated with this drug.

Co-trimoxazole (combination of sulfamethoxazole and trimethoprim): is associated with rare but serious side effects, e.g. Stevens–Johnson syndrome, toxic epidermal necrolysis, bone marrow depression (neutropenia, thrombocytopenia and purpura) and agranulocytosis.

9) I

10) A

11) D

12) E

Note
Interleukin 2: is mainly produced by Th1 (T-helper 1) cells. It activates T and NK cells and supports their growth.

Interleukin 4: is produced by Th2 cells and promotes lymphocyte growth. It is also involved in IgE responses.

Interleukin 6: is produced by Th2 cells and macrophages. It promotes B-cell growth and antibody production.

Interleukin 10: is produced by CD4 cells and activated macrophages. It inhibits the production of IL-1, IL-6, interferon-γ, tumour necrosis factor-α (TNF-α) and antigen presentation.

Interleukin 12: is produced by macrophages and monocytes. It augments Th1 responses and induces interferon-γ.

Interferon-α: is produced by leucocytes. It causes immune activation and modulation following viral infection.

Transforming growth factor β: is produced by platelets. It is immunoinhibitory but also stimulates tumorigenesis, angiogenesis and fibrosis.

13) F

14) E

15) H

16) A

Note
Different lung volumes and definitions

- The volume of air that is inspired or expired with each normal breath is the tidal volume (500 mL).
- The total lung capacity is the amount of air after maximal inspiration (6 litres in males and 4.7 litres in females).
- Inspiratory reserve volume is approximately 3 litres (maximum volume of air that can be inspired over the inspiration of tidal volume).
- Expiratory reserve volume is approximately 1.2 litres (maximum volume of air that can be expired after the expiration of the tidal volume).
- The volume of gas that remains in the lungs after maximal expiration is the residual volume (1200 mL).
- The volume of gas that remains in the lungs after normal expiration (2.3 litres) is called the functional residual capacity (expiratory reserve volume plus the residual volume).
- Inspiratory reserve volume plus tidal volume = inspiratory capacity.
- The volume of breathing apparatus that does not participate in the gas exchange is called the dead space (total 300 mL). It can be the anatomical dead space (volume of gas in conducting airways = 150 mL) or the physiological dead space (the volume of lung tissue that does not participate in the gas exchange = 150 mL).
- Functional residual capacity and residual volume cannot be measured by spirometry.

17) G

18) D

19) J

20) A

Note
ECG changes in the following conditions

Acute myocardial infarction: ST elevation, Q waves present.

Atrial fibrillation: irregular R–R interval and no P waves on the ECG.

Complete heart block: there is no relationship between P and QRS complexes. There is also a bradycardia.

Hyperkalaemia: tall T waves.

Hypokalaemia: U waves.

Left bundle-branch block: wide QRS complexes, poor R waves in the anterior septal leads.

Pulmonary embolism: S1Q3T3 (S wave in lead 1, Q wave in lead 3, inverted T wave in lead 3) and tachycardia.

Right bundle-branch block: right ventricular strain.

Ventricular bigemini: alternate QRS complexes wide >0.12 seconds.

Wolff–Parkinson–White syndrome: short P–R interval, delta wave and wide QRS complexes.

21) G

22) E

23) I

24) F

Note
Chemical teratogens and effects

Phenytoin: facial defects, learning disability (fetal hydantoin syndrome).

Sodium valproate: spina bifida and heart defects.

Trimethadione: intrauterine growth retardation, cleft palate, microcephaly, urogenital, gastrointestinal and heart defects (fetal trimethadione syndrome).

Lithium: Ebstein anomaly.

Thalidomide: Limb defects.

Warfarin: chondrodysplasia punctata, microcephaly, recurrent intracerebral haemorrhage. The risk is highest during the first trimester (approximately 10% during the first trimester and 3–5% during the second and third trimesters).

Amphetamines: cleft lip and palate.

Cocaine: microcephaly, behavioural abnormalities, growth restriction and gastroschisis.

Alchohol: fetal alchohol syndrome, short philtrum, maxillary hypoplasia, short palpebral fissures, heart defects and learning disability.

Isotretinoin: severe dysmorphic features including cleft palate, small jaw, small abnormally shaped ears, mandibular hypoplasia, heart defect and thymic aplasia. These together are called retinoic embryopathy.

Carbamazepine: neural tube defects.

25) D

26) H

27) J

28) A

Note
The various terminologies used to describe skin lesions

Ecchymosis: large confluent area of purpura.

Erosion: partial loss of skin.

Macule: flat circumscribed lesion.

Petechia: small dot-like macules of blood.

Purpura: large macule or papule of blood.

Plaque: large elevated flat lesion.

Papule: small, circumscribed, palpable lesion (<0.5 cm).

Ulcer: total loss of epidermis and dermis.

29) G

30) H

31) D

32) **C**

Note
Endometrial changes are divided into three phases

– Proliferative phase or follicular phase.
– Secretory phase – luteal phase.
– Menstrual phase or menstruation.

The endometrium is prepared for implantation during the menstrual cycle and, in the absence of fertilization, menstruation occurs. The changes occur throughout the cycle in the functionalis layer while the basalis remains static and regenerates the functionalis every month.

During the proliferative phase, increasing levels of oestrogen cause proliferation of the stromal tissue and endometrial glands (glands are elongated and epithelial cells contain little glycogen).

During the secretory phase, the glycogen and mucus are secreted from the endometrial glands under the influence of progesterone (glands become tortuous and have large lumens due to increased secretory activity). At this stage the spiral arteries extend into the superficial layer of the endometrium.

Menstruation occurs in the absence of fertilization and implantation. The corpus luteum degenerates and as a result oestrogen and progesterone levels fall. This causes involution of the endometrium (spiral arteries constrict and rupture) leading to shedding of the apoptosed (dead) endometrium.

33) **A**

34) **D**

35) **I**

36) **F**

Note
Ultrasound findings

Cephalocele: protrusion of a cystic structure through a calvarial bone defect. The most common site is the occipital region.

Cerebral ventriculomegaly: ventricular dilatation >10 mm. It can be unilateral or bilateral and can be associated with congenital anomalies or may be an acquired condition due to infection and haemorrhage.

Arnold–Chiari malformation: the cerebellum is banana-shaped plus there is obliteration of the cisterna magna.

Choroid plexus cysts (fluid trapped within the spongy layer of cells): the incidence is 1% during second trimester scans. In most cases, it is a normal finding and usually disappears by 24–28 weeks of pregnancy.

They are detected on routine second trimester ultrasound examination. This may be an isolated finding or can be associated with chromosomal anomalies (trisomy 18).

Holoprosencephaly: partially or completely fused thalami or ventricles (single ventricle), absence of cavum septum pellucidum, dysgenesis of corpus callosum and associated midline facial abnormalities (with a single eye and midline proboscis in the region of the nose). It is associated with trisomy 21.

Miller–Dieker syndrome: it is associated with lissencephaly, cardiac defects, microcephaly, polydactyly and facial anomalies.

Schizencephaly: the cerebral hemispheres contain cerebrospinal fluid (CSF)-filled abnormal clefts extending from the subarachnoid space to the lateral ventricle.

Walker–Warburg syndrome: it is associated with lissencephaly, ventriculomegaly, midline anomalies, microphthalmia and cataract.

Dandy–Walker syndrome: the appearance is that of a cyst within the posterior fossa due to gross enlargement of the cisterna magna. The cerebellar vermis is deficient and there is wide separation of the cerebellar hemispheres.

37) E

38) B

39) D

40) E

Note
Elevation of tumour markers/hormones and the respective tumours for which they are used

Choriocarcinoma: βhCG levels.

Dysgerminoma: lactate dehydrogenase (usually elevated).

Endodermal sinus tumour: α-fetoprotein.

Mixed germ cell tumours: both βhCG levels and α-fetoprotein.

Granulosa cell tumour: inhibin and oestrogen (can present with precocious puberty).

Serous cystadenocarcinoma: CA-125.

Mucinous cystadenocarcinoma: CA-125 and CEA (may be elevated).

Colon cancer: CA-19.9 and CEA (carcinoembryonic antigen).

Sertoli–Leydig cell tumour: plasma testosterone and other androgens (can present with symptoms and signs of virilization).

41) F

42) A

43) G

44) D

Note

Rocky Mountain spotted fever: it is a vector-borne disease transmitted through the bite of hard ticks, the reservoir being rodents. An eschar may develop after an incubation period of 4–10 days with an associated regional lymphadenopathy. The patient presents with sudden onset of headache, fever, myalgia, with petechial maculopapular rash. The diagnosis is mainly by history and clinical symptoms. The confirmatory test is by indirect fluorescent antibody test or latex agglutination test. The drug of choice is doxycycline or tetracycline. The alternative drug is ciprofloxacin.

Q fever: it is transmitted through the bite of hard ticks and animals are the reservoir of infection. It is mainly transmitted to humans by dust or unpasteurized milk from infected cows or aerosols. The symptoms are non-specific with fever, headache and myalgia. They could also develop pneumonia, hepatitis and other organs can be involved. Doxycycline is used for its treatment.

Epidemic typhus: the reservoir of infection is humans and it is transmitted by the human body louse. The patients present with fever, headache and myalgia after an incubation period of 1–3 weeks. Subsequently, a macular eruption appears which becomes purpuric. After 1 week they may develop meningoencephalitis. It can involve other organs and may even cause acute renal failure. Doxycycline is used for its treatment.

Endemic typhus or murine typhus: the reservoir of infection is rodents and it is spread by rat fleas to humans. The symptoms are similar to epidemic typhus but less fatal.

45) A

46) F

47) H

48) I

Note

Both *Trichomonas vaginalis* and bacterial vaginosis cause an offensive vaginal discharge. Gonorrhoea is transmitted sexually and caused by

Neisseria gonorrhoeae. In women, the cervix is usually the first site of infection. The other organs that can be involved are the rectum and the eyes. Women can pass this infection to their newborn infant during delivery and it can cause conjunctivitis (ophthalmia neonatorum). Chancroid is a bacterial infection caused by *Haemophilus ducreyi* (Gram-negative streptobacillus). In women the most common location for ulcers is on the labia majora and they are usually painful. Foreign travel is nearly always involved as the disease is found primarily in developing countries. Syphilitic ulcers are classically single and non-painful. Primary herpes simplex is characterized by flu-like symptoms followed by painful vulval ulcers with inguinal lymphadenopathy.

49) A

50) G

51) B

52) E

Note
Ovulation age = fertilization age or menstrual age minus two weeks. The morula enters the uterus after three days and transforms into a blastocyst. It then comes into contact with the endometrium on the fifth or sixth day. Subsequently, it burrows into the endometrium and comes into contact with the maternal circulation at the end of the second week. This is when implantation bleeding occurs and this coincides with the timing of the menstrual period.

Second week post ovulation – implantation
Third week post ovulation – germinal disc
Fourth week post ovulation – folding of the embryo
Fifth to eighth week post ovulation – organogenesis.

The pharyngeal and branchial arches appear in the fourth week of gestation in the head and neck region. The lower respiratory system develops during week four. The bones appear in the limb bud during the fifth week. Ossification of the long bones begins at the end of week seven and is present in all long bones by 12 weeks. Secondary ossification centres appear in the epiphysis from 34–38 weeks at the distal end of the femur and the proximal end of the tibia. Ossification of the vertebraes begins during the embryonic period and ends at the age of 25 years.

53) I
Women with PCOS can present with the above-mentioned symptoms plus infertility and are at high risk of developing hypertension, diabetes, endometrial hyperplasia and endometrial cancer.

54) E

This is drug-induced hyperprolactinaemia.

55) C

The diagnosis is an imperforate hymen and the young girl typically presents with cyclical monthly lower abdominal pain. The treatment is cruciate incision on the hymen to make a passage for the blood to flow. It is usually done under general anaesthesia.

56) H

57) I

58) J

59) F

60) B

Primary amenorrhoea is defined as the absence of menses at the age of 16 years in the presence of normal growth and secondary sexual characteristics.

The causes of primary amenorrhoea include:
Gonadal dysgenesis
Mullerian agenesis: absence of uterus, cervix, vagina or all of them
Imperforate hymen or transverse vaginal septum
Hypothalamic amenorrhoea
Congenital adrenal hyperplasia
Androgen insensitivity syndrome
Pituitary diseases.

Secondary amenorrhoea is defined as the absence of menses for more than three menstrual cycles or six months in women who have previously menstruated.

The causes of secondary amenorrhoea include:
Polycystic ovarian syndrome
Asherman syndrome
Premature ovarian failure
Post chemotherapy
Post pelvic radiotherapy.

61) I

Most of the high-grade cervical intraepithelial lesions (pre-cancerous lesions – CIN II and CIN III) are caused by HPV types 16 and 18.

62) H

63) D
Herpes simplex type I causes both oral and genital lesions. The lesions are usually painful.

64) C

65) A
Transitional epithelium lines both bladder and ureters.
Brenner's tumour of the ovary is also lined by transitional epithelium.

66) E
The labia majora also contain sweat and sebaceous glands.

67) G

68) B

Note
- The endocervix is lined by columnar epithelium.
- Bartholin glands are lined by cuboidal to columnar epithelium.
- The lateral surface of the labia minora and clitoris are lined by stratified squamous epithelium with sweat and sebaceous glands (except on the glans).
- The ovarian surface is lined by a single layer of cuboidal cells (germinal epithelium) with dense connective tissue beneath called tunica albuginea. It is made up of the cortex (contains follicles and corpora lutea) and a vascular medulla.

69) B
The other lateral branches include the renal, middle suprarenal and the ovarian arteries.

70) E
The lumbar artery is also a dorsal branch of the aorta and supplies the muscles of the back, vertebrae and the nerves.

71) A
The coeliac trunk also supplies the oesophagus, duodenum and liver.

72) C
The superior mesenteric artery is also a ventral branch of the aorta and supplies the bowel up to the transverse colon.

73) F

74) F

75) E

76) A

Note
Routes of transmission

The infectious diseases that are transmitted by the faeco-oral route include:
Hepatitis A
Hepatitis E
Cholera
Shigella
Salmonellosis
Polio
Rota virus.

The diseases that are transmitted by the transplacental route include:
HIV
Hepatitis B
Syphilis.

The diseases that are transmitted by the droplet or respiratory route include:
Measles
Mumps
Rubella
Whooping cough
Tuberculosis
Chicken pox
Influenza.

The diseases that are transmitted by sexual route include:
HIV
Hepatitis B
Gonorrhoea
Syphilis
Trichomonas vaginalis
Genital warts
Chlamydia
Herpes simplex type I and 2.

The diseases that are transmitted by blood and blood products include:
HIV
Hepatitis B
Cytomegalovirus.

The diseases that are transmitted by organ transplantation include:
Cruetzfeldt–Jacob disease
Cytomegalovirus infection.

77) D
Vasopressin is an antidiuretic hormone and causes water retention (by altering the permeability in the collecting ducts in the kidney).

78) D
Oxytocin causes contractions of the myoepithelial cells (allowing release of milk) and myometrial cells (labour).

79) E
Thyrotrophin-releasing hormone (TRH) stimulates thyroid-stimulating hormone (TSH) production from the anterior pituitary.

80) A
Corticotrophin-releasing hormone (CRH) stimulates adrenocorticotrophic hormone (ACTH) production from anterior pituitary.

4. Practice EMQs II: Questions

1–4)

Options

A.	Cytoplasm
B.	Nucleolus
C.	Nucleus
D.	Mitochondria
E.	Golgi apparatus
F.	Endoplasmic reticulum
G.	Ribosomes
H.	Phagosomes
I.	Lysosomes
J.	Centrioles

Instructions: Select the most appropriate organelle for each of the functions referred to below from the list of options. Each option may be used once, more than once or not at all.

1) RNA production

2) Oxidize proteins, fats and carbohydrates into energy

3) Digestion of unwanted endogenous material

4) Digestion of unwanted phagocytosed exogenous material

5–8)

Options

A.	Vitamin A
B.	Vitamin D
C.	Vitamin K
D.	Vitamin E
E.	Vitamin B_1
F.	Vitamin B_6
G.	Folic acid
H.	Vitamin B_5
I.	Vitamin B_{12}
J.	Vitamin C

Instructions: Select the most appropriate vitamin for each of the functions referred to below from the list of options above. Each option may be used once, more than once or not at all.

5) Antioxidant

6) One carbon transfers

7) Hydroxylation of proteins in collagen

8) Coenzyme A formation

9–12)

Options

A.	Cystic fibrosis
B.	Familial hypercholesterolaemia type IIa
C.	Familial hypercholesterolaemia type IV
D.	Familial hypercholesterolaemia type 1
E.	Hereditary non-polyposis coli
F.	Lesch–Nyhan syndrome
G.	Maple syrup urine disease
H.	Porphyrias
I.	Sickle cell disease
J.	Xeroderma pigmentosa

Instructions: Select the most appropriate disease from the above list of options for each of the symptoms and signs referred to below. Each option may be used once, more than once or not at all.

9) Tendon xanthomas

10) Self-mutilation

11) Seizures

12) Basal cell carcinoma

13–16)

Options

A.	Chylomicrons
B.	LDL and chylomicrons
C.	LDL
D.	LDL and VLDL
E.	Fatty acid
F.	Triacylglycerols
G.	VLDL
H.	VLDL and chylomicrons
I.	VLDL, LDL and chylomicrons
J.	Cholesterol

Instructions: From the options above, select the most appropriate lipoprotein class that is raised for each of the hyperlipidaemias listed below. Each option may be used once, more than once or not at all.

13) Inherited hyperlipidaemia type 1

14) Inherited hyperlipidaemia type 2A

15) Inherited hyperlipidaemia type 2B

16) Inherited hyperlipidaemia type 4

17–20)

Options

A.	Arrhenoblastoma
B.	Basal cell carcinoma
C.	Burkitt lymphoma
D.	Breast carcinoma
E.	Basaloid carcinoma
F.	Follicular lymphoma
G.	Lung adenocarcinoma
H.	Neuroblastoma
I.	Ovarian carcinoma
J.	Retinoblastoma

Instructions: Select the most appropriate cancer for each of the proto-oncogenes referred to below from the list of options. Each option may be used once, more than once or not at all.

17) Mutation of *K-ras*

18) *HER-2/neu* gene

19) Amplification of *c-myc*

20) Translocation of *c-myc* from chromosome 8 to chromosome 14

21–24)

Options

A.	Becker muscular dystrophy
B.	Duchenne muscular dystrophy
C.	Glucose-6-phosphate dehydrogenase deficiency
D.	Hypogammaglobulinaemia
E.	Haemophilia A
F.	Haemophilia B
G.	Retinitis pigmentosa
H.	Ocular albinism
I.	Vitamin D-resistant rickets
J.	X-linked ichthyosis

Instructions: Select the most appropriate X-linked disease for each of the abnormalities referred to below from the list of options. Each option may be used once, more than once or not at all.

21) Factor IX reduced

22) Corneal opacities

23) Reduced steroid sulphatase enzyme

24) Patchy depigmentation of the retina

25–28)

Options

A.	Albinism
B.	Glucose-6-phosphate dehydrogenase deficiency
C.	Galactosaemia
D.	Gaucher disease
E.	Tay–Sachs disease
F.	Hurler syndrome
G.	Hunter syndrome
H.	Niemann–Pick disease
I.	Phenylketonuria
J.	Pentosuria

Instructions: Select the most appropriate genetic disease for each of the enzyme abnormalities mentioned below from the list of options. Each option may be used once, more than once or not at all.

25) Tyrosinase

26) Glucocerebrosidase

27) Hexosaminidase A

28) Sphingomyelinase

29–32)

Options

A.	Ascorbic acid
B.	Biotin
C.	Calciferol
D.	Carotenes
E.	Cobalamin
F.	Folic acid
G.	Niacin
H.	Pyridoxine
I.	Riboflavin
J.	Thiamine

Instructions: Select the most appropriate vitamin deficiency from the list of options above for the conditions mentioned below. Each option may be used once, more than once or not at all.

29) Pernicious anaemia

30) Rickets

31) Pellagra

32) Beri-beri

33–36)

Options

A.	Drug therapy to increase the excretion of copper
B.	Replacement of the hormone – cortisone
C.	Replacement of the hormone – calcitonin
D.	Replacement of the hormone – thyroxine
E.	Replacement of the enzyme – tyrosinase
F.	Phenylalanine-restricted diet
G.	Phenylalanine-free diet
H.	Replacement of vitamin – calciferol
I.	Removal of the disease – thyroidectomy

Instructions: Select the most appropriate therapy or treatment from the list of options above for the genetic diseases mentioned below. Each option may be used once, more than once or not at all.

33) Congenital adrenal hyperplasia

34) Congenital cretinism

35) Phenylketonuria

36) Wilson disease

37–40)

Options

A.	Coarctation of aorta
B.	Conn syndrome
C.	Cushing syndrome
D.	Essential hypertension
E.	Pre-eclampsia
F.	Pregnancy-induced hypertension
G.	Phaeochromocytoma
H.	Raised intracranial hypertension
I.	Renal hypertension
J.	White coat hypertension

Instructions: Match the clinical and biochemical features described below with the list of hypertensive disorders mentioned above. Each option may be used once, more than once or not at all.

37) Hypertension, hypokalaemia, alkalosis plus normal glucose tolerance test

38) Paroxysms of hypertension associated with anxiety, palpitation and glucose intolerance

39) Hypertension associated with easy bruising, proximal myopathy and glucose intolerance

40) On examination, one would be able to feel the radial pulse earlier than the femoral pulse

41–44)

Options

A.	Acute appendicitis
B.	Acute intermittent porphyria
C.	Cholecystitis
D.	Cystitis
E.	Duodenal ulcer
F.	Gastric ulcer
G.	Meckel diverticulum
H.	Pancreatitis
I.	Pyelonephritis
J.	Renal colic

Instructions: Select the single most likely diagnosis from the list of options above for the clinical presentations described below. Each option may be used once, more than once or not at all.

41) A 36-year-old woman presents with epigastric pain that is relieved by intake of food

42) A 38-year-old morbidly obese woman presents with epigastric pain (radiating through to the back), nausea and vomiting. She is in her second pregnancy (34 weeks pregnant) and gives a history of gallstones

43) A 26-year-old woman presents with pain in the right iliac fossa, nausea and vomiting. On abdominal examination there is rebound tenderness and guarding in that area

44) An 18-year-old woman presents to A&E with pain in the right loin and a spiking temperature, and she generally feels unwell. She is currently 16 weeks pregnant and gives a history of recurrent suprapubic pain during this pregnancy. Her urine dipstick is positive for proteins and nitrates

45–48)

Options

A.	Absence of A and B antigens with presence of anti-A and anti-B antibodies
B.	Absence of A and B antigens with absence of anti-A and anti-B antibodies
C.	Presence of A antigen on red blood cells with serum anti-A antibodies
D.	Presence of B antigen on red blood cells with serum anti-B antibodies
E.	Presence of A antigen on red blood cells with serum anti-B antibodies
F.	Presence of B antigen on red blood cells with serum anti-A antibodies
G.	Presence of both A and B antigen with serum anti-A and anti-B antibodies
H.	Presence of both A and B antigens with absence of anti-A and anti-B antibodies
I.	Presence of anti-H antibodies
J.	Absence of anti-H antibodies

Instructions: Match the blood groups given below with the presence or absence of antigens on red blood cells and antibodies in serum of individuals listed above. Each option may be used once, more than once or not at all.

45) Blood group A

46) Blood group B

47) Blood group AB

48) Blood group O

49–52)

Options

A.	β-Thalassaemia
B.	Diaphragmatic hernia
C.	Cytomegalovirus infection
D.	Congenital toxoplasmosis
E.	Fetal tachyarrhythmia
F.	Idiopathic
G.	Parvovirus infection
H.	Rhesus isoimmunization
I.	Twin-to-twin transfusion
J.	Sacrococcygeal teratoma

Instructions: Select the most appropriate cause for hydrops from the list of options above for each case described below. Each option may be used once, more than once or not at all.

49) A 31-year-old Asian woman is referred to the day assessment obstetric unit at 36 weeks' gestation in view of the large-for-date uterus on examination. Her blood sugar is normal and an urgent growth scan reveals single intrauterine fetus with signs of hydrops fetalis. She is rhesus positive with no antibodies to the red blood cells. She is known to have sickle cell trait and her partner is negative for sickle cell trait or disease

50) A 36-year-old white woman presents to the day assessment unit with reduced fetal moments. She complains of a fever, rash and arthralgia. A growth scan of the fetus at 28 weeks shows features of hydrops. She is rhesus negative with no antibodies to red blood cells. She has normal haemoglobin on the electrophoresis test

51) A 40-year-old African–Caribbean woman, who has not been booked, undergoes an emergency caesarean section at 36 weeks for fetal distress. The baby is cyanosed at birth and needs immediate intubation by the paediatricians. On auscultation of the heart the baby was found to have dextrocardia

52) A 32-year-old Turkish woman who is gravida 3 para 2 comes to antenatal clinic on follow-up visit at 32 weeks' gestation. She had a fetal loss at 36 weeks in her previous pregnancy. Her current growth scan shows features of hydrops in fetus. She is rhesus negative with antibodies to red blood cells

53–56)

Options

A.	Intramuscular anti-D immunoglobulin injection (50 IU)
B.	Intramuscular anti-D immunoglobulin injection (100 IU)
C.	Intramuscular anti-D immunoglobulin injection (250 IU)
D.	Intramuscular anti-D immunoglobulin injection (500 IU)
E.	Intramuscular anti-D immunoglobulin injection (250 IU) plus a Kleihauer test
F.	Intramuscular anti-D immunoglobulin injection (500 IU) plus a Kleihauer test
G.	Intramuscular anti-D immunoglobulin injection (2500 IU)
H.	Intramuscular anti-D immunoglobulin injection (5000 IU)
I.	Subcutaneous anti-D immunoglobulin injection (500 IU)
J.	Anti-D injection not required

Instructions: Select the most appropriate anti-D immunoglobulin requirements from the list of options above for each case described below. Each option may be used once, more than once or not at all.

53) A 22-year-old woman comes with a history of mild per vaginal bleeding. She is 8 weeks pregnant by her last menstrual period and an ultrasound scan shows a viable intrauterine pregnancy. She is rhesus negative with no red cell antibodies

54) A 25-year-old woman comes to the Early Pregnancy Assessment Unit (EPAU) at 8 weeks pregnancy with abdominal pain. An ultrasound scan shows a left-sided ectopic pregnancy for which she undergoes a left salpingectomy. She is rhesus negative with no red cell antibodies

55) A 41-year-old woman comes to antenatal clinic for routine follow-up. She is currently 34 weeks pregnant with a low lying placenta. Her blood group is B rhesus negative with no red cell antibodies

56) An 18-year-old girl undergoes a second trimester medical termination of pregnancy at 14 weeks' gestation. She is discharged home and subsequently found to be blood group A rhesus negative with no red cell antibodies

57–60)

Options

A.	Stage Ia
B.	Stage Ib
C.	Stage Ic
D.	Stage IIa
E.	Stage IIb
F.	Stage IIIa
G.	Stage IIIb
H.	Stage IIIc
I.	Stage IVa
J.	Stage IVb

Instructions: Match the following findings on the histology given below with the uterine staging options mentioned above. Each option may be used once, more than once or not at all.

57) Endometrial adenocarcinoma confined to the uterus but involving more than half the myometrium

58) Endometrial adenocarcinoma involving less than half the myometrium and cervical stroma

59) Endometrial adenocarcinoma invading the rectal mucosa

60) Endometrial adenocarcinoma involving inguinal lymph nodes

61–64)

Options

A.	Ankylosing spondylitis
B.	Goodpasture syndrome
C.	Hashimoto thyroiditis
D.	Hodgkin disease
E.	Leprosy
F.	Polymyositis
G.	Polycystic kidney disease
H.	Rheumatoid arthritis
I.	Systemic lupus erythematosus
J.	Schizophrenia

Instructions: Select the most appropriate HLA linkage given below for each of the diseases mentioned above. Each option may be used once, more than once or not at all.

61) HLA-B27

62) HLA-B5

63) HLA-DR4

64) HLA-DR5

65–68)

Options

A.	Aortic stenosis
B.	Aortic regurgitation
C.	Bacterial endocarditis
D.	Mitral stenosis
E.	Mitral regurgitation
F.	Mitral valve prolapse
G.	Pericardial effusion
H.	Pulmonary hypertension
I.	Peripartum cardiomyopathy
J.	Tricuspid regurgitation

Instructions: Select the most appropriate cardiovascular pathology for each of the cases referred to below from the list of options. Each option may be used once, more than once or not at all.

65) A 36-year-old woman who had a normal vaginal delivery 3 weeks ago attends A&E with a history of a gradual onset of fever. On examination she has painful red spots over her palms and early diastolic murmur was heard over the left parasternal area. An echocardiogram shows vegetations near the aortic valve

66) A 30-year-old woman who had an uneventful vaginal delivery 6 weeks ago comes to A&E with increasing shortness of breath. On cardiovascular examination the apical impulse is diffuse and displaced downwards. A chest radiograph shows cardiomegaly

67) A 50-year-old woman had a radical hysterectomy for endometrial cancer 2 months ago. Subsequently she received pelvic radiotherapy. Three months later she attends A&E with a decrease in her urine output and shortness of breath. Her ECG shows a low-voltage complex and a chest radiograph shows a globular heart with clear lung fields

68) A 25-year-old pregnant woman attends the obstetric day assessment unit with palpitations. A cardiovascular system examination shows mid-systolic click with late systolic murmur on cardiac auscultation

69–72)

Options

A.	Chronic obstructive pulmonary disease (COPD)
B.	Chronic sinusitis
C.	Cirrhosis of the liver
D.	Congestive cardiac failure
E.	Diabetic acidosis (ketoacidosis)
F.	Mild asthma
G.	Nephrotic syndrome
H.	Pregnancy with hyperventilation
I.	Renal calculi
J.	Recurrent excessive vomiting in early pregnancy

Instructions: Match each of the acid–base responses given below with the clinical conditions mentioned above. Each option may be used once, more than once or not at all.

69) Respiratory alkalosis

70) Respiratory acidosis

71) Metabolic alkalosis

72) Metabolic acidosis

73–76)

Options

A.	α_1-Adrenergic receptor
B.	α_2-Adrenergic receptor
C.	β_1-Adrenergic receptor
D.	β_2-Adrenergic receptor
E.	Histamine (H_1) receptor
F.	Histamine (H_2) receptor
G.	Muscarinic–cholinergic receptor
H.	Nicotinic–cholinergic receptor
I.	Dopamine receptors
J.	Opioid receptors

Instructions: Select the most appropriate receptor from the above list of options for the agonist actions described below. Each option may be used once, more than once or not at all.

73) Agonist action causing vasoconstriction

74) Agonist action causing bronchodilatation

75) Agonist action causing an increase in heart rate

76) Agonist action causing a decrease in heart rate

77–80)

Options

A.	3β-Hydroxysteroid dehydrogenase
B.	5α-Reductase
C.	11β-Hydroxylase
D.	11-Hydroxysteroid dehydrogenase
E.	17,20-Desmolase
F.	17α-Hydroxylase
G.	17β-Hydroxysteroid dehydrogenase
H.	20,22-Desmolase
I.	18-Hydroxylase
J.	21-Hydroxylase

Instructions: Select the most appropriate enzyme from the above list of options for the steps involved in hormone synthesis. Each option may be used once, more than once or not at all.

77) Converts pregnenolone to 17-hydroxypregnenolone

78) Converts androstenedione to testosterone

79) Converts 17-hydroxyprogesterone to 11-deoxycortisol

80) Converts dehydroepiandrosterone to androstenedione

4. Practice EMQs II: Answers

1) B

2) D

3) I

4) I

Note
Endoplasmic reticulum: is involved in protein synthesis. The nucleolus helps in ribosome and RNA production. The ribosome catalyses peptide bond formation and secretion.

5) D

6) G

7) J

8) H

Note
Other names for different vitamins:

Vitamin A – retinol
Vitamin D – calciferol
Vitamin K – menaquinone
Vitamin E – tocopherol
Vitamin B_1 – thiamine
Vitamin B_6 – biotin
Vitamin B_5 – pantothenic acid
Vitamin B_{12} – cobalamin
Vitamin C – ascorbic acid.

9) B

10) F

11) G

12) J

Note

Familial hypercholesterolaemia type IIa: in this condition, there is a genetic defect in the low-density lipoprotein (LDL) receptor gene. It is associated with high levels of LDL. The clinical manifestations include tendon xanthomas, xanthelasma and early onset ischaemic heart disease with a positive family history of coronary artery disease in the young. The treatment is mainly lifestyle modification, reduced dietary cholesterol intake and drugs, e.g. statins (simvastatin, pravastatin, atorvastatin – HMG-CoA reductase inhibitors), niacin and bile acid sequestrants.

Lesch–Nyhan syndrome: is an X-linked recessive condition in which there is deficiency of the enzyme hypoxanthine–guanine phosphoribosyl transferase (HGPRT), leading to excess uric acid levels in the body as well as increased excretion of uric acid in the urine. The clinical manifestations include the triad of hyperuricaemia, behavioural and cognitive impairment (e.g. self-mutilation) and central nervous system dysfunction. The treatment is mainly symptomatic, e.g. the drug allopurinol is used for gout and lithotripsy for renal calculi.

Maple syrup urine disease: is an autosomal recessive disorder caused by deficiency of the branched-chain α-ketoacid-dehydrogenase complex (BCKDH) resulting in high levels of leucine, isoleucine and valine in the blood as well as the urine. The clinical manifestations include vomiting, seizures, opisthotonus, pancreatitis, ketoacidosis leading to coma and death in infancy or childhood. Infants present with sweet-smelling urine similar to maple syrup. The treatment involves a diet low in leucine, isoleucine and valine.

Xeroderma pigmentosa: is an autosomal recessive disorder in which there is a defect in DNA repair (the body is unable to repair the damage caused by ultraviolet rays to the skin). The clinical manifestations include severe sunburn, freckles, dark spots on the skin, blisters and premature ageing of the skin. This can lead to basal cell carcinoma, malignant melanoma or squamous cell carcinoma. The treatment involves avoiding exposure to the sun. The skin manifestations can be treated with isotretinoin, fluorouracil or cryotherapy.

13) A

14) C

15) D

16) G

Note

Inherited hyperlipidaemia type I: is caused by a deficiency of lipoprotein lipase, which results in increased chylomicron levels in the blood.

Inherited hyperlipidaemia type 2A: incidence is 1 in 1000 people and it is an inherited disease that leads to high blood cholesterol levels (LDL). The amount of cholesterol is regulated by the liver and it uses receptors or docking sites to perform this function. Inheritance of an abnormal gene on the docking site from one or both the parents leads to this condition.

A person can be asymptomatic to start with and, at the other extreme, can manifest with coronary artery disease. The cholesterol can deposit at different sites, such as knuckles of the hand, eyelids, elbows and Achilles tendons. A combination of drugs is usually necessary to reduce the blood cholesterol levels, e.g. statins and niacins.

Inherited hyperlipidaemia type 2B: is caused by LDL-receptor deficiency and increased ApoB (apoprotein B). This results in an increase in very-low-density lipoprotein (VLDL) and LDL. The treatment is statins, niacin and fibrates.

Inherited hyperlipidaemia type 3: is associated with increased intermediate-density lipoprotein (IDL) and the drug of choice for treatment is fibrates.

Inherited hyperlipidaemia type 4: is associated with increased VLDL and the serum is characteristically turbid. The drug of choice is either fibrate or niacin.

17) G

18) D

19) H

20) C

Note
Proto-oncogene

Alteration of the normal gene by mutation leads to the formation of an oncogene. This can contribute to the development of cancer (the mutated proto-oncogene, now called an oncogene, can cause the cell to multiply in an unregulated manner in the absence of normal growth signals). Different functions in the cell may be undertaken by the proto-oncogene, e.g. signals that lead to cell division (code for proteins that help to regulate cell growth and differentiation) and apoptosis (programmed cell death).

21) F

22) J

23) J

24) H

Note
Haemophilia A: is an X-linked recessive disorder caused by deficiency of factor VIII. The treatment is regular infusion of recombinant factor VIII.

Haemophilia B: is an X-linked recessive disorder caused by deficiency of factor IX. The treatment is regular infusion of recombinant factor IX.

X-linked ichthyosis: is caused by inherited deficiency of steroid sulphatase. The clinical manifestations include scaling of the skin, particularly involving the extensor surfaces of the body. The symptoms are better during the summer. The treatment is symptomatic and supportive.

Ocular albinism: is divided into three types and can present with nystagmus, strabismus, colour blindness, night blindness and loss of hearing. The treatment is symptomatic, e.g. visual aids for refractive errors such as myopia and hyperopia, and surgery for conditions like strabismus and nystagmus.

25) A

26) D

27) E

28) H

Note
Albinism: is usually autosomal recessive although other forms of inheritance exist (autosomal dominant and X linked). It is characterized by the absence of pigmentation of the skin and eyes and is associated with visual disorders.

Gaucher disease: is an autosomal recessive disease caused by deficiency of the enzyme glucocerebrosidase. Its clinical manifestations include anaemia, thrombocytopenia, neurological symptoms and hepatosplenomegaly. It can be diagnosed prenatally by the absence of enzyme activity in cultured amniotic fluid cells.

Tay–Sachs disease: is an autosomal recessive condition caused by deficiency of the enzyme hexosaminidase A. The clinical manifestations include severe physical retardation and learning disability, with degenerative neurological changes (onset before 1 year of age and early death at the age of 2–4 years), and a cherry-red spot on the macula is seen on fundoscopy. It can be diagnosed prenatally by the absence of enzyme activity in cultured amniotic fluid cells.

Niemann–Pick disease: is an autosomal recessive condition caused by deficiency of the enzyme sphingomyelinase. The clinical manifestations include severe neurological symptoms, a cherry-red spot on the macula and hepatosplenomegaly. It can be diagnosed prenatally by the absence of enzyme activity in cultured amniotic fluid cells.

29) E

30) C

31) G

32) J

Note
Ascorbic acid (vitamin C): deficiency causes scurvy.

Biotin: deficiency causes dermatitis.

Calciferol (vitamin D): deficiency causes rickets in children and osteomalacia in adults.

Carotenes (vitamin A): deficiency causes xerophthalmia.

Cobalamin: is vitamin B_{12}.

Folic acid: deficiency causes megaloblastic anaemia.

Niacin: deficiency causes pellagra (characterized by dermatitis, diarrhoea and dementia).

Pyridoxine: is vitamin B_6.

Riboflavin (vitamin B_2): deficiency causes dermatitis and cheilosis.

Thiamine (vitamin B_1): deficiency causes beri-beri (heart failure and neurological effects).

33) B
The deficient production of glucocorticoids and excess formation of androgens in congenital adrenal hyperplasia (CAH) give rise to symptoms of failure to thrive and also ambiguous genitalia at birth. The main form of replacement therapy is cortisone.

34) D
Congenital cretinism is congenital hypothyroidism and thus replacement of thyroxine is the treatment.

35) G
The manifestations of phenylketonuria in an untreated child include severe learning disability, microcephaly, decreased melanin production, blonde hair and blue eyes. The enzyme phenylalanine hydroxylase

cannot be replaced, so removal of phenylalanine from diet is the main modality of treatment.

36) A
In Wilson disease, there is excess accumulation of copper in the body. The use of drugs such as penicillamine (chelating agent) to increase the excretion of the copper may be helpful in the treatment.

37) B
Conn syndrome is due to an excess of mineralocorticoid (aldosterone), resulting in increased excretion of potassium which causes hypokalaemia.

38) G
Phaeochromocytoma is also associated with a history of headaches, vomiting, palpitation and sweating.

39) C
Cushing syndrome is due to an excess of glucocorticoids and, in addition to the above findings, it is associated with excessive weight gain, purple skin striae and acne.

ACTH-induced Cushing syndrome causes hypokalaemic alkalosis and hypertension together with glucose intolerance.

Increased glucocorticoid excess from a pituitary cause is called Cushing disease (there is no hypokalaemia).

40) A
This clinical sign is called radiofemoral delay.

41) E
The pain in the epigastric region may be aggravated or relieved by the intake of food. This kind of pain is usually related to a peptic ulcer; in a gastric ulcer the epigastric pain is aggravated by food and in a duodenal ulcer the epigastric pain is relieved by food. The pain may improve with antacids and H_2-receptor antagonists (ranitidine).

42) H
Pancreatitis is rare during pregnancy and women usually present in the third trimester. A high index of suspicion is important during pregnancy as clinical signs may be masked due to gravid uterus. Raised serum amylase levels (can be >1000 U/L) would further help in making a diagnosis. The management is supportive unless the woman develops serious complications.

43) A
The presenting complaint in appendicitis is usually classic as described above. The pain usually starts in the umbilical region before localizing to

the right iliac fossa. It is associated with clinical signs of peritonism and a serum inflammatory marker (white cell count) may be raised.

It usually presents in the first two trimesters of pregnancy with atypical presentation in late pregnancy due to the size of the gravid uterus. The abdominal pain may be higher up on the right side of the abdomen, e.g. women may present with pain in the subhepatic region as the caecum and appendix are pushed up due to the gravid uterus in late pregnancy. So a high index of suspicion is important as delay in diagnosis can lead to increased morbidity (perforation).

44) I
Recurrent cystitis is common during pregnancy and can lead to pyelonephritis if untreated. The patient may need admission for investigations (midstream urine for culture and sensitivity, blood tests for full blood count, blood culture and renal function tests), hydration, temperature control and intravenous antibiotics.

45) E

46) F

47) H

48) A

Note
ABO blood groups were discovered by Landsteiner. A, B, AB and O blood are the major phenotypes and can be determined by an isoagglutination reaction, which can be seen by the naked eye as clumping of red cells.

49) F
This is idiopathic as no specific cause is found for hydrops.

50) G

51) B

52) H

Note
The causes of hydrops can be immune (associated with rhesus incompatibility, anti-Kell antibodies and anti-Fya antibodies), non-immune (severe congenital heart disease, fetal arrhythmias, twin-to-twin transfusion, homozygous α-thalassaemia, parvovirus B19 infection, diaphragmatic hernia and congenital adenomatoid malformation of the

lung, chromosomal anomalies, renal anomalies and placental chorioangioma) and idiopathic (no specific cause is found).

53) J

The sensitization is less likely with bleeding or miscarriage before 12 weeks' gestation and therefore anti-D is not required.

Anti-D should be considered if bleeding and pain are excessive and the woman is near to 12 weeks' gestation. It is also recommended if a termination or evacuation of retained products of conception is performed before 12 weeks' gestation. Anti-D (250 IV) is given if miscarriage, bleeding or termination occurs after 12 weeks from gestation.

54) C

55) D

56) C

Note

Read the RCOG guideline on use of anti-D immunoglobulin for Rh prophylaxis (revised May 2002):

- The administration of anti-D immunoglobulin injection is recommended to rhesus-negative women following delivery. A Kleihauer test may be helpful to determine if any extra fetomaternal haemorrhage has occurred and identifies the need for additional anti-D dose.
- Anti-D immunoglobulin should be given after any sensitizing event before delivery (e.g. external cephalic version, abdominal trauma, antepartum haemorrhage) and after abortion/termination.
- NICE recommends 500 IU of anti-D immunoglobulin to non-sensitized rhesus-negative women at 28 and 34 weeks of pregnancy.

57) C

58) E

59) I

60) J

Note

FIGO staging of endometrial cancer

Stage Ia: endometrial cancer confined to the endometrium.

Stage Ib: endometrial cancer confined to the uterus but involving less than half of the myometrium.

Stage Ic: endometrial cancer confined to the uterus but involving more than half the myometrium.

Stage IIa: endometrial cancer involving cervical glands but not the stroma (confined to the uterus and cervix).

Stage IIb: endometrial cancer involving cervical stroma (confined to the uterus and cervix).

Stage IIIa: endometrial cancer involving the uterine serosa, tubes, adnexa and positive peritoneal cytology.

Stage IIIb: vaginal metastasis.

Stage IIIc: endometrial cancer involving pelvic and para-aortic nodes.

Stage IVa: endometrial cancer involving the bladder or rectum.

Stage IVb: distant metastasis including intra-abdominal and inguinal lymph nodes.

61) A

62) G

63) H

64) C

Note
Diseases and HLA association

Goodpasture syndrome: HLA-DR7, DR8
Hodgkin disease: HLA-B18
Leprosy: HLA-B8
Polymyositis: HLA-A1, B8, DR3
Systemic lupus erythematosus: HLA-B8, DR3
Schizophrenia: HLA-A28.

65) C
The treatment for bacterial endocarditis is intravenous antibiotics for 4–6 weeks based on the blood culture sensitivity results.

66) I
A patient with peripartum cardiomyopathy usually needs admission to an intensive care unit, review by a cardiologist, diuretics, angiotensin-converting enzyme (ACE) inhibitors/angiotensin receptor blockers (ARBs) and β blockers.

67) G

Radiotherapy can lead to retroperitoneal fibrosis (bilateral ureteral fibrosis), which can in turn lead to renal failure and uraemic pericardial effusion. In this case an echocardiogram confirms cardiac tamponade and therefore the patient needs peri-cardiocentesis.

68) F

Mitral valve prolapse: if a woman is asymptomatic then she can be left alone; however, if she does become symptomatic she will need a mitral valve repair (balloon valvuloplasty)

69) H

Respiratory alkalosis due to hyperventilation is physiological. The arterial blood gases (ABGs) can show the following: pH 7.54, PCO_2 2.5 kPa, PO_2 12 kPa and HCO_3^- 22 mmol/L.

70) A

In respiratory acidosis, the ABGs can show pH 7.25, PCO_2 7.8 kPa and HCO_3^- 22 mmol/L.

71) J

In metabolic alkalosis, the ABGs can show pH 7.56, PCO_2 5.5 kPa and HCO_3^- 33 mmol/L.

72) E

In metabolic acidosis, the ABGs can show pH 7.24, PCO_2 5.5 kPa and HCO_3^- 17 mmol/L.

73) A

Drug agonists acting on the α_1-receptors include adrenaline, noradrenaline and isoprenaline.

Drug agonists acting on the α_2-receptors cause sedation and hypotension.

74) D

Drug agonists acting on the β_2-receptors cause bronchodilatation, uterine relaxation (tocolytic agents such as ritodrine, salbutamol and terbutaline) and vasodilatation. These also have some β_1-receptor actions.

75) C

Drug agonists acting on β_1-receptors cause an increase in the heart rate, e.g. dobutamine and dopamine.

76) G

Drug agonists acting on muscarinic receptors can also cause bronchoconstriction and increase in gut motility and secretions, while agonist action on nicotinic receptors causes contraction of the striated muscle.

77) F

The enzyme 17α-hydroxylase is also involved in the conversion of progesterone to 17-hydroxyprogesterone.

78) G

The enzyme 17β-hydroxysteroid dehydrogenase is also involved in the conversion of dehydroepiandrosterone to 5-androstenediol.

79) J

The enzyme 21-hydroxylase is also involved in the conversion of progesterone to deoxycorticosterone. This is the most common enzyme deficiency leading to congenital adrenal hyperplasia.

80) A

The enzyme 3β-hydroxysteroid dehydrogenase is also involved in conversion of pregnenolone to progesterone, of 17-hydroxypregnenolone to 17-hydroxyprogesterone.

Suggested reading: the steroid hormone synthesis cycle.

Reference:

Murray RK, Redwell VW, Beuder D, et al. *Harper's Illustrated Biochemistry*, 28th edn. Maidenhead: McGraw-Hill Medical, 2009.